GET WELL

AN A–Z OF NATURAL MEDICINE FOR EVERYDAY ILLNESSES

Russell Setright's

GET WELL

AN A–Z OF NATURAL MEDICINE FOR EVERYDAY ILLNESSES

Russell Setright, B.App.Sc., N.D., D.B.M.

ATRAND PTY LTD
Suite 2, 77 Willoughby Road,
Crows Nest, NSW, 2065

Copyright © Russell Setright 1990
Reprinted 1991
ISBN 0-908272-22-7
Printed in Australia by Griffin Press

Note:
This book is for educational purposes only. It is not designed to
treat or diagnose disease or injuries to the body. The author,
publisher and printer accept no responsibility for such use.

Never discontinue your practitioner's medication without their
advice and consult your practitioner if suffering from any disease, injury or illness.

THE AUTHOR

RUSSELL SETRIGHT
B.App.Sc., N.D., D.B.M., H.D.,

Naturopath, Herbalist,
and Clinician.

Russell Setright is one of Australia's most well-known and leading naturopaths.

Since the 1980s he has been promoting Natural Therapies throughout Australia, Singapore and Malaysia through numerous radio and television shows. He also writes regular newspaper and magazine columns. His current shows include a weekly talk-back program on Radios 2GB and 2CA Canberra, and regular weekly segments on various country and interstate radio stations. He has appeared on a weekly television segment on Vision TV, Toowoomba, Living in Brisbane and Good Morning Sydney.

Russell is the Naturopathic Director at Blackmores and runs the Blackmores Naturopathic Clinic and Research Centre at Chatswood, Sydney, and is the editor of "Clinically Speaking".

Russell Setright trained in industrial chemistry and worked in this field for 15 years and rose to the position of General Manager. Stress and poor diet, and smoking led to a heart attack. He began studying nutrition, herbal medicine and naturopathy and restored himself to good health.

He gained a Diploma in Naturopathy and Herbal Medicine with honours. Russell is a Fellow of The Society of Natural Therapists and Researchers, a Fellow of the Academy of Natural Therapies, a member of NHAA, ATMS, ANTA, Government Registered Naturopath (NT), Vice Chairman ANTA (NSW) and National Practitioner Liaison Officer for ANTA. He has professional qualifications in First Aid and is an instructor/examiner with St John Ambulance Australia.

Russell spends much of his leisure time helping others in his position as National Flag Officer Medics in the Royal Volunteer Coastal Patrol Australia. He is a captain and runs the Coastal Patrol/St John Water Ambulance, 'Blackmores Rescue', at weekends on a voluntary basis. He believes there is a need for more understanding between practitioners of different health care disciplines, and he is in a unique position to promote this.

FOREWORD

Russell Setright's book is a very valuable and sensible Australian book covering nutrition, herbs, lifestyle and dietary changes; information that we all need.

This book extracts knowledge from the experience gained from years of contact with the public through his clinic, TV and radio programs. The book is a ready-reckoner for health problems. It is able to be used as a day-to-day reference (manual) for health. It covers most problems, most methods of treatment, yet pays strict attention to the human body's requirements and dosages of therapeutic substances.

What the reader can learn from this book is gained from referenced clinical experience. Applying the hard data towards this work is very similar to Dr Setright's approach to his very successful appearances on radio programs in Australia and his involvement with Blackmores Naturopathic Clinics and Research Centres.

Dr Alan McLeay, MB, BS (Syd.)

ACKNOWLEDGEMENTS

There are a number of people I wish to thank for their help. Firstly, my dear, departed mother, who, when I made the decision to move out of corporate management and become a Naturopath, was the only person to stand by me and give me encouragement. Without her support I would not have been able to complete the many years of study needed to qualify as a Naturopath and, indeed, write this book.

To my family, who supported and stood by me, putting up with the countless hours I sat around the dining room table with reference books and my computer. To my secretary, Pauline Garside, who has been of enormous help and support. To Dr Alan McLeay, whose counsel I have often sought through the years and who has been kind enough to write the Foreword in this book. To Marcus Blackmore, whose unselfish and charitable actions towards his fellow human being, and his belief that all people should have the right to actively participate in all forms of medicine available to them in order to improve their own health, has been an inspiration to me to forge ahead. To my good friends and tutors, Ross Mack, Principal of the Academy of Natural Therapies in Queensland and Denis Stewart, Principal of the Southern Cross Herbal School, for their support throughout the years. To Professor Don Napper for whom I worked as a research assistant more than twenty years ago. It was he who taught me that the answer to any seemingly impossible quest could be solved tomorrow, if you do not give up today. To Catherine Warne for help with the Guide to Herbs Used in this Book, and to Barbara McGregor and Paul Callinan for their contribution to Reasons for Supplementing with Vitamins and Minerals.

Finally, my thanks go to the thousands of listeners of my radio and television programmes to whom I have spoken over the years. It was their questions which influenced my selection of topics in this book.

RUSSELL SETRIGHT

CONTENTS

PART 1
Nutrition   1
The Six Basic Nutrients   1
Recommended Dietary Allowance   9
Dietary inadequacies of Schoolchildren   15
Dietary inadequacies of Adults   17

PART II
The A–Z of Common Illnesses
Acne or Acne Vulgaris   20
Ageing Spots   21
AIDS (see Immune System)
Alcohol   23
Allergies   24
Alzheimer's Disease (see Memory)
Analgesics   26
Antioxidants   27
Arthritis   28
Asthma   30
Athletes and Regular Exercisers   31
Babies' Problems   32
Back Pain   33
Bad Breath   35
Bedsores   35
Bites and Stings   36
Blood Pressure   38
Bowel Polyps   40
Bran   40
Bronchitis   42
Bruising or Bruises   43
Burns   43
Calcium   44
Cancer   47
Caffeine   50
Candida   50
Chilblains   52
Children and Multi vitamins   53
Cholesterol   54
Cigarette Smoking   56
Cold Hands and Feet   58
Cold Sores   59

Colon Care   60
Common Cold and Flu   61
Constipation   61
Cracking Skin   62
Cramps   63
Crohn's Disease   64
Cystitis .   65
Dandruff and Itchy Scalp   66
Diabetes Mellitus   67
Diarrhoea   68
Diverticulitis   69
Dry Skin   70
Epilepsy   71
Eyes and Night Vision (see Night Vision)
Food Allergies (see Allergies)
Fasting   73
Fluid Retention   74
Gallstones   75
Garlic   77
Gout or Crystal Arthritis   78
Hawthorn   79
Hayfever   81
Headaches   82
Heart Disease   84
Healthy Nails   86
Hepatitis (see Liver)
Herpes (see Cold Sores)
How to Lose Weight   86
Hyperactivity and Children   87
Hypoglycaemia   88
Immune System and Viral Infections   89
Impotency   91
Indigestion and Dyspepsia   92
Insomnia   93
Leg Pain   94
Leg Ulcers (see Bed Sores)
Liver Health   95
Medication and Drugs (see Prescribed Drugs)
Memory   97
Menopause   98
Menstruation   99
Migraine   100

Mouth Ulcers   102
Multiple Sclerosis (see Immune System)
Nails (see Healthy Nails)
Night Vision and Eyesight   102
Osteoarthritis   103
Osteoporosis   104
Painful Menstruation (see Menstruation)
Pre Menstrual Tension   105
Pregnancy   106
Prescribed Drugs   108
Prostate Problems   108
Psoriasis (see Skin Disorders)
Raynaud's Syndrome (see Cold Hands and Feet)
Rheumatoid Arthritis (see Arthritis)
Ringing in the Ears (see Tinnitus)
Sinusitis   109
Skin Disorders   110
Smoking (see Cigarette Smoking)
Sore Throat   111
Strains and Sprains   111
Stress   112
Tinnitus and Vertigo   113
Travel Sickness   114
Varicose Veins   115
Vertigo (see Tinnitus)
Warts   115
Weight Loss   116
Zinc   120

PART III
Guide to Herbs Used in This Book   **122**

PART IV
Vitamins — Minerals and Their Uses   **143**

PART V
Understanding Medical Terminology   **157**

References
Index

INTRODUCTION

Australia is probably one of the most spectacular and yet under-rated countries. When I last travelled overseas I was surprised to find people in Europe and the USA still believe that Australia is a land of 'boxing' kangaroos wandering our main streets. In fact, in lifestyle, culture and climate we are very similar to the west coast of North America.

When in friendly conversation you mention to a North American that Australia has sheep stations comparable in area to that of the state of Texas and that before the first world war, we had one of the world's largest populations of wild horses, you will find you are looked on in disbelief.

I wonder how well we Australians know Australia? We all read books and learn our history mainly from overseas and our ethnic backgrounds have also made their mark. Australia is a country of many mixed cultures and people and we still have to realise that this is Australia and we are unique.

Just think for a moment about one of our customs.

It is Christmas and the thermometer reaches 35°C. Mum, the grandparents, and an assortment of children are all lined up around a magnificently decorated fir tree covered in artificial snow and shimmering tinsel. This reminds us that only last night a fat, jolly white bearded man dressed in a head to toe red flannel suit climbed down our chimney with a merry HO! HO! HO! and filled the stockings full of toys for all the good boys and girls.

On Christmas day we all sit down to a large helping of HOT roast turkey, baked potatoes, vegetables followed by a course of mum's hot steamed pudding and custard. It's good to remember the old times back 'home' but just how far should we go? Our fashions, the latest foods, and even our lifestyle, are dictated to Australians from such faraway places as London, Paris, New York, and Rome. We need to remember we are Australians with our own local traditions and lifestyle.

With the introduction of processed foods and medications, and the addition of artificial colourings, flavourings and preservatives, our daily lifestyle has been slowly eroded. We are now all looking for the way to good health and improved quality of life with the use of natural medicines such as herbs. We wish to exclude such non-foods as artificial colouring, flavourings, and preservatives. We seek, with an ever-increasing awareness of the environment, to reduce pollution both of water and the atmosphere and strive to achieve a never-ending improved physical and mental fitness. If we are successful we are on the way to gaining our ultimate goals of health, fitness, and long life.

Of the number of books written about herbs, diet and nutrition there has not been a book written that considers the special problems of the Australian climate, diet and environment.

Throughout this book I will endeavour to cover the different aspects of human life and the special requirements living in our wonderful and very different island continent, Australia.

If we sit back and think for a moment about our own lifestyle, most of us will realise that as individuals, our own requirements for the simple things of life such as the food we eat, the type of house we live in, and the car we drive, are all part of our make-up. It is this make-up that to a certain degree decides how well we can expect to be for the rest of our lives.

We are what we eat and how we live. Most illnesses that Australians suffer are caused directly by their lifestyle. If we do the right thing many illnesses can be prevented.

Australia can be a hard, unforgiving land if we do not learn to live with it. Problems like the highest rate of skin cancer in the world, one of the highest consumption rates of beer per head of population, and the ever-increasing level of pollution in our cities are slowly leading the average Australian into poor health.

We will look now at how we can improve our health with a little care and thought for our daily routines.

What Type of Lifestyle Have You?

There are a number of things that have enormous effects on our lifestyle. Let's first look at stress. Are we under stress or aren't we? This is an interesting question and one that I am asked a lot.

Just imagine that we are back in the time of the cavemen and women. We know from the cave paintings and drawings that the diet of the cave man consisted of the odd mastodon stew, some herbs and fresh fruit straight off the tree (not stored for some months), good unfertilised greens with the occasional yam and lots of fresh, clean, unpolluted water. AHHHH! That sounds good doesn't it? There certainly doesn't seem to be any stress there. What a life!

Wait a minute! What about the mastodon stew? If I remember my anthropolgy, man, at that time, was only around the same size as he is today and the odd mastodon weighed many tonnes. So here we have it, man on one side armed to the teeth with a pointed stick and some rocks to throw (we'll call him Fred) and on the other side we have 10 tonnes of muscle-bound fury with two enormous sword-like tusks ready to do battle.

Do you think that a little stress may be developing here? I know that if I were placed in the same situation, I would be under stress and would probably turn vegetarian on the spot. However, the history books tell us Fred didn't! If this is so, how did he do it? The answer is stress.

This overwhelming problem of modern day man is the very thing that saved the day for Fred. But how could stress possibly help? The answer is the biological role that stress plays. This biological role is a kind of built-in attack and defence mechanism, for as Fred moved in on his prey, his body was undergoing a number of chemical changes.

Fred's muscles would need more power and oxygen. His breathing and heart rate would increase along with an increase in blood pressure, which would push that river of life, his blood, through his body. Fred was now ready to fight or run. He was at his physical and emotional peak. There is one factor I should mention. When Fred took on this beast and if all went well and he won the fight, there was still the possibility that he may have suffered the odd scratch. Don't worry, the Almighty already thought of that and, at the same time, the clotting ability of Fred's blood was increased. This was done by increasing the level of fat in the blood stream which would help plug the scratch.

Once the battle was over, Fred would then take his prize back home to receive a hero's welcome, wind down and have a well-earned, long, stress-free rest. Fred could function very well under these conditions. A period of short term stress, the satisfaction of a job well done, the praise and thanks of his family and periods of stress-free rest to enjoy.

Let's now look at modern day Fred.

Fred is still subjected to a number of stresses. Although he may no longer need to fight the wild beast for his very existence, there

is a new more dangerous problem: psychological stress. This
form of stress, mainly unknown to Fred of old, is built up by
such problems as economic pressures or competition in our daily
lives, either at work or at school. We are constantly striving to
meet the goals that have been set by others, the noise of modern
day life, the deadlines, queues and interruptions, all push us to
the breaking point. If you drive a car then you are again subjected to even greater stress.

Let's now look at the hypothetical lifestyle of Mr and Mrs
Jones. It is a beautiful sunny Monday morning. The first rays of
sunlight break through the window-pane into the Jones' bed-
room, pushing aside the darkness, ready for a new day. Outside,
the streets are quiet with the exception of the tinkling of milk
bottles and the distant barking of a dog. What an ideal, stress-
free picture this makes. But, just as suddenly as those first rays of
sunlight kissed the covers on the Jones' bed, a loud and irritating
noise smashes the silence. It is the alarm on the bedside table
that has just heralded the start of the Jones' day. The alarm is
usually set at this time so that a number of regimental duties can
now be performed. Mr and Mrs Jones have planned this time
carefully. There has to be enough time to jump out of bed,
shower, eat the maximum of food in the minimum of time (this
usually means a cup of black coffee gulped down with a slice of
toast), jump into the family car and off to work. Again, the time
was planned so that they arrive at work exactly on time. They
wouldn't want to waste one minute of their precious leisure time
by arriving at work one minute early, would they?

Well, if everything goes as planned Mr and Mrs Jones will
arrive at their respective destinations on time. As the Jones' drive
up the street a terrible thing happens. The traffic lights that are
green have suddenly turned red. The Jones' car is third from the
lights and in front of them they have an elderly gentleman,
wearing a top hat, driving an old Rover. Directly behind them is
a Morris Minor with five ladies all wearing white bowlers' hats.
The lights change, and horror of horrors, the first car doesn't
move for thirty seconds. This, of course, holds the second car up
for another thirty seconds. By this time the car behind them is
tooting the horn and the level of stress for the Jones' is on the
rise.

They have now been robbed of over two minutes of their
allocated time and they have to make it up. Fighting for every
foot of road like a general planning a battle, they manoeuvre

their car from lane to lane keeping one foot on the brake and other foot on the accelerator so they can prevent the driver on their right or left from claiming their 4 metres of ground.

I have spent some time watching the attitudes of different drivers as they approach the toll gates of the Sydney Harbour Bridge. Some people have one arm out the window banging on the roof while the other is driving. Having looked at his watch, twisted up his face in frustration he began to pound the steering wheel, not unlike the battle cry of a crazed ape who beats on his chest before the kill. This type of behaviour slowly, minute by minute, raises the blood pressure and increases stress levels.

The Jones', having experienced these pressures and stress, have arrived at work to find their parking place taken and now they are really in the mood for a day's work! If all their efforts in the preceeding battle were wasted and they are indeed five minutes late, then they will either be hauled on the mat before the boss, have their pay adjusted or hear some appropriate remark from their peers such as, 'They always come late and never get into any trouble. They must have something going with the boss.'

All of this really doesn't help them wind down from their already stress-filled morning. Lunchtime usually comes around and after having washed they are ready to eat. Usually, they have enough time left to gulp down their junk food lunch and wash it down with a hot cup of coffee. At the same time they listen to all the latest news about whoever isn't there to defend themselves.

At last, at the end of the working day, they arrive home after another thrilling experience in the traffic. They are now in the domain of their own home. Like Fred of old in his cave, they can now rest, put the feet up and relax. But something goes wrong. Little Johnny has a social tonight and his clothes are still in the wash. Quickly, one of them gets up to attend to the clothes. There is no time to lose. It will have to be done before dinner which must be ready by 6 pm.

Mr Jones arrived home having had a day just like Mrs Jones. When she tries to relate the events and problems of her day she is cut short in her conversation with comments such as, 'You think that's bad, you should have seen what happened to me!' This, of course, only increases the frustration and instead of winding down, both end up bottling up the stress and frustrations of the day. Because of their lifestyle, Mr and Mrs Jones are in danger.

They are suffering from that all too common problem, chronic stress.

The side-effects of this long term, bottled up form of stress are almost endless. They include confusion, disturbances in sleep, irritability, increased blood pressure, heart rhythm disturbances, lowered resistance to viral infections, headaches, tense muscles. The list goes on and on. If you feel you fit into a little of the Jones' lifestyle, then you too may be at risk and a change may be required.

Most of us have already selected our goals and have committed ourselves to hire purchase, a home mortgage, and to that end are unable to change the main direction of our lives. But we can modify our lifestyles in many ways so that we can cope with the outside pressures that are placed upon us which we cannot change.

Good health and the management of stress go hand in hand. It depends on the fitness of our bodies. The first step is exercise such as walking, jogging, swimming. All of these exercises help to improve the fitness of the body by toning the muscles, increasing the flow of oxygen-rich blood through the body and improving the function of most organs in the body. We must not forget that our insides require exercise as well. The correct amount of roughage in a well-balanced diet is all part of good health. Just as your car requires the correct petrol and oil, our bodies cannot function without the correct balance of food, water, air, and exercise. A good way to make sure that you are getting the right amount of roughage is to take two or three apple fibre complex tablets each day as part of your daily plan. Because stress uses some of the micro nutrients such as vitamin B group, vitamin C and the celloid minerals potassium phosphate and magnesium phosphate more quickly, extra supplementation is required. A Naturetime Executive B Formula which includes all of the vitamins and minerals along with three very important and time-proven herbs, can help calm stressed and tired nerves.

How many people have heard the old story about the little old lady who smoked like a chimney, drank whisky out of the bottle, went out with bad men and lived to be 95 years old. When she died they had to beat her liver to death with a stick. Well, there is always the exception to the rule, isn't there, but how many of us forget the man up the street who last week, at 38 years of age, died on the squash courts from a massive heart attack. Poor Mr Jones, this is a bit close to home, isn't it? The fact is that now is the time to start listening to the old saying that tomorrow is the first day in the rest of your life and it can't be put off.

PART I
NUTRITION

Nutrition — Why is it Important?

First, what is this thing we call nutrition? All of us have seen a
never-ending number of fad diets: some to control weight, others
supposedly to stop us growing old. Where will it end? We seem to
be getting further and further away from the basics. In this
chapter, we will look at the six basic nutrients that make our food
and what part they play in our bodies.

Nutrition is not just what we eat but what we absorb from our
foods.

The Six Basic Nutrients
1 Water
2 Carbohydrates
3 Fats
4 Proteins
5 Vitamins
6 Minerals

Water

The first nutrient that we have on the list is probably the most
under-rated and yet the most important.

Did you know that your body is made up of around 70%
water? This water is needed to form blood and body fluids
without which our bodies would not be able to dissolve and carry
the essential nutrients to all parts of the body. Water is needed in
the body to help maintain the body temperature and it is also
needed to carry away the body's waste products.

The human body will die if deprived of water for only a few
days. Yes, our water supply is very important to us and the

average Australian should consume around 8 to 10 glasses of water each day in the form of foods containing water or liquids.

Carbohydrates

There are three types of carbohydrates that are important to us:

Polysaccharides: These are the most complex of the carbohydrates and they are made up from many carbohydrate units. The most common polysaccharide in our diet would be in the form of starch which is found in grains such as rice, wheat, corn. Other foods such as potatoes are another good source of complex carbohydrate.

The other carbohydrates are monosaccharides and disaccharides.

Disaccharides: These are a double sugar: sucrose, lactose, and maltose. Sucrose, or table sugar is the most widely consumed disaccharide. The average consumption of sugar in Australia is around 60kg per person per year. In these quantities sugar is a health problem, leading to heart disease and other health problems.

Monosaccharides: There are three types of monosaccharides: glucose, fructose, and galactose. Glucose is the most important monosaccharide. All other carbohydrates are either obtained from it or changed into it. The body stores glucose by changing it into glycogen which is stored in the muscles and liver. This can be easily changed back to glucose when the body requires it for quick energy.

The main function of carbohydrates is to supply the body with energy and for the formation of cellular constituents.

A lack of carbohydrate in the diet (as with some of the liquid quick weight-loss diets) can lead to the production of ketones in the body. This increase in ketones decreases the alkalinity and increases the acidity of the blood resulting in a condition known as Ketosis and metabolic acidosis. It is important to balance the diet as metabolic acidosis can be very serious.

Your carbohydrate intake should be around 60 per cent of your food intake in the form of complex carbohydrates. Eating too many monosaccharides such as table sugar is not the way to get your sugar requirement. Although it will give quick energy (because of the increased blood sugar level) these levels soon drop and leave you feeling run down and craving for more sugar. Eat fruit instead.

Fats

Fats, or lipids, furnish us with twice as much energy for our bodies than that of protein or carbohydrate. Fat is needed in our daily diet for the correct usage of fat soluble vitamins A, D, E, K.

Fat insulates our bodies giving us protection from sudden changes in temperature and at the same time protects the vital organs of the body against damage.

The average Australian consumes around 40 per cent of their total calorie intake in the form of fat. Fat is important in the diet because it gives the diet staying qualities as fat is absorbed in the body at a much slower rate than that of carbohydrate or protein. This is very important because it makes the meal satisfying, so, by having a little fat in our diets the feeling of hunger will be delayed.

There are two types of substances that give fat different flavours and textures. They are known as fatty acids, either saturated (which come mainly from animal sources) or unsaturated, including polyunsaturated fatty acids (which come from the vegetable kingdom) and are found in foods such as nuts, vegetables, and seeds. There are three essential fatty acids. They are linolenic, arachidonic, and linoleic. All are very important and because they cannot be manufactured in our bodies they must become an integral part of our daily diet.

Protein

Protein is the second most plentiful substance in our bodies next to water. Protein builds new tissue and repairs damaged cells. Protein also is needed in our bodies for the formation of hormones and enzymes which play a variety of roles in the body such as metabolism, growth, and sexual development. It is also used by the body to regulate the body's fluid level and help control the acid alkaline level.

Protein consists of around 22 amino acids which are the building blocks of protein. Protein is classified into two types: complete and incomplete proteins.

Complete proteins supply all of the 8 essential amino acids: lysine, tryptophan, phenylalanine, methionine, threonine, leucine, isoluecine, valine. Eggs are the best source of amino acids (complete proteins), followed by dairy products and meats.

Vegetarians can obtain their protein from seeds, nuts and lentils but it is best to vary the diet and obtain your dietary protein from a range of different foods. Remember eggs, dairy products, and red meats are high in cholesterol. The use of egg whites, skim milk, lean meats and fish is best.

Diet for a Healthy You

To understand about diet we must know a little of what is going on inside our bodies when we eat our food.

There is a very complex action on the food we eat by digestive enzymes such as protease, an enzyme that can break down protein and amylaze, one of the enzymes that can break down carbohydrate. These processes break the food we eat down into micro-nutrients such as amino acids (the building blocks of protein), vitamins, minerals, fats, carbohydrates. Only foods that have been broken down this way can be absorbed into the systemic system of the body.

There are a number of things that can interfere with the proper digestion and absorption of foods into our bodies. Some factors are illness, pollution, and stress. The air we breathe and the water we drink are part of our daily food intake. If these are polluted then the absorption of our food will be affected.

Heart and vascular diseases, gastric and indigestion problems are the most common problems that affect our quality of life as we grow older. We have looked at some of the problems such as stress, pollution, smoking, and lifestyle that are all critical in reducing our quality of life.

It is now time to look at the most important part of our daily life and that is what and how we eat. We, as Australians, need a diet to suit us, not bits and pieces that we have picked up from tradition or the junk foods that are tempting us around every corner. Vitamins cannot take the place of the well-balanced diet.

Diet is the cornerstone of all therapy and, unfortunately, most Australians do not recognise this.

Patients suffering from a variety of complaints such as indigestion, constipation ask 'Is there something natural that I can take to solve my problem?'

The answer is yes, but that is not the answer that I give my patient. My approach is to look at the lifestyle and diet. Too often I find that the diet is made up in one day of toast, sweetened coffee or tea, biscuits, softdrink, a meat pie or sausage roll, hot chips; cream bun; sausages or fried foods, bread, tomato sauce, and peas, mashed potato and gravy.

This is typical food for a number of working persons in Australia. These foods are high in refined carbohydrates, fat, artificial additives. Although these people gain weight, some are suffering from malnutrition, which we consider when we think of the starving children of the third-world countries.

This is not the case for the average Australian. However, with such a diet there is a possibility that some micro-nutrients, fibre and even protein may be lacking, and the daily balance of nutrients is way out. In the sample, there is far too much fat, too much cholesterol, the salt (sodium) level is too high, so is the refined sugar. Let's just look at some of the levels of nutrients in this daily diet and see what we have. I think a lot of you will be surprised.

Food substance	mg sodium
bread (two slices)	230
butter (one teaspoon)	200
meat pie	750
hot chips	150
biscuits (two sweet)	80
sausage (two)	1000
tomato sauce (2 tablespoons)	600
gravy (1 teaspoon dry mix)	300
TOTAL	3310

This level of sodium (salt) in our diet is far in excess of what the average Australian needs to maintain a healthy life. I made no allowance for salt to be added to any of the above meals.

Research has shown us that the average Australian consumes around 4000mg of sodium per day when only 200mg to 300mg of sodium is required each day by the average working Australian to maintain a healthy life.

This excess of sodium in the body can cause many problems such as increased blood pressure and increased fluid retention.

The excess sodium that has been supplied by the diet is usually excreted by the kidneys and to do this the normal fluid levels in the body are raised so that the extra sodium can be kept in solution and the normal fluid sodium concentration in the body can be met. Because of this the blood volume in the arteries is increased followed by a corresponding increase in the blood pressure. This increase in blood pressure is returned to normal when the excess sodium is excreted from the body. However, there are about 30 per cent of Australians that are generally sensitive to excess sodium in their diets. These people could have permanently elevated blood pressure which could result in premature heart diseases, if they continually eat salty foods.

You may ask, 'If we can't eat the type of diet shown above, what can we eat?'

To answer that question I have put together a basic daily diet containing all of the basic food groups of dairy products, meat, fish, eggs, fruit, and vegetables.

Fad diets and eating habits, if not advised by your practitioner, can be dangerous to your health. If you reduce your intake of calories to less than 450 per day you slow down the production of thyroxin in the body and lower your metabolic rate and this lowering of metabolic rate could remain even after resuming normal eating habits. The problem then is that the weight just comes back again.

Let us now look at a diet that would suit the average Australian.

A LARGE GLASS OF FRESH WATER FIRST THING EACH MORNING

BREAKFAST

Glass orange or pineapple juice (unsweetened)

Poached eggs with 1 slice of kibble bread, lightly spread with butter (3 times per week only).

and/or

1 serve of natural muesli, wheat cereal. Add natural fruit to sweeten, some unprocessed bran or oat bran, skim milk or soy milk, no sugar. A little honey may be used now and then.

1 cup of herbal tea.

MORNING TEA

1 medium-sized apple

LUNCH

Salad. (If you are not able to take this type of lunch with you to work and you can buy your lunch, then order salad sandwiches)

Include in your salad: lettuce leaves, cucumber slices, stick celery, tomato, grated carrot and cottage cheese, slices beetroot, pineapple, natural yoghurt; 1 cup herbal tea;

AFTERNOON TEA

1 glass vegetable juice; or 1 glass fruit juice;

DINNER

Glass of water, nut meat or lentils with salad or vegetables Don't overcook vegetables, stir-fry with a little olive oil or steamed is best. Use herbs to enhance the flavour. or grilled chicken (no skin) or steamed or grilled fish with lemon or grilled veal and side salad. Add a little cold pressed oil to apple cider vinegar, garlic and some herbs to taste.

Alternate this with steamed vegetables including at least 4 to 5 different vegetables both green and yellow

DESSERT

Use natural fruit and yoghurt.

Your water intake should be between 6 to 8 glasses per day. This may include herbal tea.

Acid alkaline food balance

All food which is digested in the body leaves a residue. This residue can be either acid, neutral, or alkaline. The body requires an excess or reserve of alkaline residue foods in the diet to maintain good health. If you eat too many foods that leave an acid residue, then a condition known as acidosis can result when there is a depletion of the reserve supply of alkali in the tissue and blood of the body.

The normal, or natural, ratio of alkaline to acid in the average healthy Australian is about 80 per cent alkaline to 20 per cent acid. This ratio is important in the maintenance of a healthy body and the resistance to disease.

The following is a list of the main foods which are either acid, neutral, or alkaline-forming foods.

Acid-forming foods

* OYSTERS	RICE
* FISH	WHOLE WHEAT
* VEAL ORGAN MEATS	CHEESE
LIVER	LENTILS
MOST GRAINS	OATMEAL
CHICKEN	PEANUTS & MOST NUTS
EGGS	

* most acid-forming foods in list

Alkaline-producing foods

* APRICOTS	CARROTS
* SOYBEANS	BEANS
* FIGS	POTATOES
BUCKWHEAT	ORANGES
LEMONS	CELERY
ASPARAGUS	BANANAS
BRAZIL NUTS	CABBAGE
LETTUCE	APPLES
ALMONDS	

* most alkaline foods in list
MILK, BUTTER AND COLD PRESSED VEGETABLE OILS ARE NEAR NEUTRAL

10 Food Rules

1 Do not eat acid-residue foods with starchy foods
2 Eat only natural foods
3 Avoid artificial colourings and additives
4 Eat most foods raw (uncooked or unprocessed)
5 Eat 80 per cent alkaline-producing food
6 Do not eat and drink at the same time
7 Take your time over meals and chew your food well
8 Plan your meals and mealtimes
9 Do not add salt or processed condiments to your meal. Use natural herbs, apple cider vinegar, and so on to add extra flavour
10 Enjoy your meal and remember, it's good to be healthy.

Recommended Dietary Allowance (RDA) Recommended Dietary Intake (RDI)

For a healthy body there is no substitute for a well-balanced diet and we all should be looking closely at the food we eat. Most of us today, because of our rushed lifestyle, unfortunately don't eat as well as we would like. Even if we did, the quality of the food may well be lacking in the essential minerals and vitamins required for healthy life.

In 11 mid-western states in the USA a 1000 crop samples were taken, and a decline in mineral levels of up to 68 per cent were noted over a four-year period. The question must be asked, 'How good is the quality of our food in comparison with that of our forebears?'

Indeed we are not getting enough from our average diet to meet the RDA levels in some nutrients. Further examples of this can be shown by investigations reported in the *American Journal of Clinical Nutrition,* 37, 1983, showing the dietary patterns of healthy pregnant women, even on a balanced diet, didn't have adequate amounts of some essential nutrients. For example, the healthy middle class North American women surveyed in the study were found to have lower levels of zinc intake, with the average only receiving 56 per cent of the RDA figure.

Worldwide studies involving people in all age groups and socioeconomic backgrounds, have shown nutritional deficiencies are common and the need for vitamin and/or mineral supplements is growing just so the RDA recommended dietary allowance can be maintained.

Stress, illness, pollution, menstruation, pregnancy, lactation, age, use of medication and increased activity, play a very important role in deciding whether or not supplements to diet are necessary and, if so, how much?

The RDA gives a figure below which known and tested deficiency symptoms would show up. If our diet was to contain less than 30mg of vitamin C, then in a short time the disease scurvy would become evident. No allowance was made in the RDA for high stress or other illnesses when working out the dietary allowance. The RDA really is a minimum allowance for persons in good health under ideal conditions.

If we look at the Australian Health Survey 1977–78, conducted by the Australian Commonwealth Government Department of Statistics, we would see that approximately 45 per cent of the Australian population suffer one or more chronic conditions. This means that nearly 50 per cent of the Australian population, at any given time, does not fit into the criteria for measuring the Recommended Dietary Allowance.

We should not be looking at the minimum levels of vitamins and minerals but the optimum daily intake needed to compensate for our lifestyle and environmental pollution.

Dr Linus C. Pauling, Nobel Laureate, Professor of Chemistry, states that the optimum daily intake of vitamin C for most human adults is between 2300 to 9000 mg and not that of 45 mg per day as stated in the RDA.

If we live a stress-free life without illness, have plenty of exercise and sleep, together with well-balanced diet without medication, and our environment is free from pollution, smog, cigarette smoke and car exhaust fumes, then we do not need supplements.

Reasons for supplementing with vitamins and minerals

1 Poor digestion
    Even when your food intake is good, inefficient digestion can limit your body's intake of vitamins. Some common causes of inefficient digestion are not chewing for long enough and eating too quickly. Both of these result in larger than normal food particle-size, too large to allow complete action of digestive enzymes. Many people with dentures are unable to chew as efficiently as those with a full set of original teeth.

2 Hot coffee, tea, and spices
    Habitual drinking of liquids that are too hot, or consuming an excess of irritants such as coffee, tea or pickles and spices can cause inflammation of the digestive linings, resulting in a drop in secretion of digestive fluids and poorer extraction of vitamins and minerals from food.

3 Alcohol
    Drinking too much alcohol is known to damage the liver and pancreas which are vital to digestion and metabolism. It can also damage the lining of the intestinal tract and adversely affect the absorption of nutrients, leading to sub-clinical malnutrition. Regular heavy use of alcohol increases the body's needs for the B group vitamins, particularly thiamine,

niacin, pyridoxine, folic acid and vitamin B12, A and C as well as the minerals zinc, magnesium and calcium. Alcohol affects availability, absorption and metabolism of nutrients.

4 Smoking
Smoking tobacco is an irritant to the digestive tract and increases the metabolic requirements for vitamin C, all else being equal, by at least 30% above the non-smoker. Smoking is known to cause heart disease.

5 Laxatives
Overuse of laxatives can result in poor absorption of vitamins and minerals from food, by hastening the intestinal transit time. Paraffin and other mineral oils increase losses of fat soluble vitamins A, E and K. Other laxatives used to excess can cause losses of minerals such as potassium, sodium and magnesium.

6 Fad diets
Bizarre diets that miss out on whole groups of foods can be seriously lacking in vitamins. Even the popular low fat diets, if taken to an extreme, can be deficient in vitamins A, D and E. Vegetarian diets, which exclude meat and other animal sources must be very skilfully planned to avoid vitamin B12 deficiency, which may lead to anaemia.

7 Overcooking
Lengthy cooking or re-heating of meat and vegetables can oxidise and destroy heat susceptible vitamins such as the B group, C, and E. Boiling vegetables leaches the water soluble vitamins B group and C as well as many minerals. Light steaming is preferable. Some vitamins, such as vitamin B6 can be destroyed by irradiation from microwaves.

8 Food storage
Freezing food containing vitamin E can significantly reduce its levels once defrosted. Foods containing vitamin E exposed to heat and air can turn rancid. Many common sources of vitamin E, such as bread and oils are nowadays highly processed, so that the vitamin E content is significantly reduced or missing totally, which increases storage life but can lower nutrient levels. Vitamin E is an antioxidant which defensively inhibits oxidising damage to all tissues. Other vitamin losses from food preserving can include vitamin B and C.

9 Convenience foods
A diet overly dependent on highly refined carbohydrates, such as sugar, white flour and white rice, places greater demand on additional sources of B group vitamins to process these carbohydrates. An unbalanced diet contributes to such conditions as irritability, lethargy, and sleep disorders.

10 Antibiotics
Some antibiotics, although invaluable in fighting infection, also kill off friendly bacteria in the gut, which would normally be producing B group vitamins to be absorbed through the intestinal walls. Such deficiencies can result in a variety of nervous conditions, therefore it may be advisable to supplement with B group vitamins when on a lengthy course of broad spectrum antibiotics.

11 Food allergies
The omission of whole food groups from the diet, as in the case of individuals allergic to gluten or lactose, can mean the loss of significant dietary sources of nutrients such as thiamine, riboflavin or calcium.

12 Crop nutrient losses
Some agricultural soils are deficient in trace elements. Decades of intensive agriculture can overwork and deplete soils, unless all the soil nutrients, including trace elements, are regularly replaced. In one USA Government survey, levels of essential minerals in crops were found to have declined by up to 68% over a four-year-period in the 1970s.

13 Accidents and illness
Burns lead to a loss of protein and essential trace nutrients such as vitamins and minerals. Surgery increases the need for zinc, vitamin E an other nutrients involved in the cellular repair mechanism. The repair of broken bones will be retarded by an inadequate supply of calcium and vitamin C and conversely enhanced by a full dietary supply. The challenge of infection places high demand on the nutritional resources of zinc, magnesium and vitamins B5, B6 and zinc.

14 Stress
Chemical, physical and emotional stress can increase the body's requirements for vitamins B2, B5, B6, and C. Air pollution increases the requirements for vitamin E.

15 PMT
Research has demonstrated that up to 60% of women suf-

fering from symptoms of premenstrual tension, such as headaches, irritability, bloatedness, breast tenderness, lethargy and depression can benefit from supplements of vitamin B6.

16 Teenagers

Rapid-growth spurts such as in the teenage years, particularly in girls, place high demands on nutritional resources to underwrite the accelerated physical, biochemical and emotional development in this age group.

17 Pregnant women

Pregnancy creates higher than average demands for nutrients, to ensure healthy growth of the baby and comfortable confinement for the mother. Nutrients which require increasing during pregnancy are the B group, especially B1, B2, B3, B6, folic acid and B12, A, D, E and the minerals calcium, iron, magnesium, zinc and phosphorus.

18 Oral contraceptives

Oral contraception can decrease absorption of folic acid and increase the need for vitamin B6 and possibly vitamin C, zinc and riboflavin. Approximately 22% of Australian women aged 15 to 44 are believed to be on the pill at any one time.

19 Light eaters

Some people eat very sparingly, even without weight reduction goals. USA dietary surveys have shown that an average woman maintains her weight on 7560 kilojoules per day, at which level her diet is likely to be low in thiamine, calcium and iron.

20 The elderly

The aged have been shown to have a low intake of vitamins and minerals, particularly iron, calcium and zinc. Folic acid deficiency is often found, in conjunction with vitamin C deficiency. Fibre intake is often low. Riboflavin (B2) and pyridoxine (B6) deficiencies have also been observed. Possible causes also include impaired sense of taste and smell, reduced secretion of digestive enzymes, chronic disease and, maybe, physical impairment.

21 Lack of sunlight

Invalids, shiftworkers and people whose exposure to sunlight may be minimal, can suffer from insufficient amounts of vitamin D, which is required for calcium metabolism, without which rickets and osteoporosis (bone thinning) has been observed. Ultraviolet light is the stimulus to vitamin D formation in skin. It is blocked by cloud, fog, smog, smoke, ordinary window glass, curtains and clothing. The maximum recommended daily supplement of vitamin D is 400 IU.

22 Bio-individuality
Wide fluctuations in individual nutrient requirements from the official recommended average vitamin and mineral intakes are common, particularly for those in high physical demand vocations, such as athletes and manual labour, taking into account body weight and physical type.

23 Athletes
Athletes consume large amounts of food and experience considerable stress. These factors affect their needs for B group vitamins, vitamin C and iron in particular. Tests on Australian Olympic athletes and A-grade football players have shown wide-ranging vitamin deficiencies.

Signs of an inadequate diet

Body part	Signs	Cause	Treatment
Face	Moonface	Prednesone therapy	—
	Oedematous (swollen)	Protein deficiency	Amino acids, protein
	Pale	Iron deficiency	Iron phosphate, B12, folic acid
	Dark skin over cheeks and under eyes (malar pigmentation)	Inadequate B group of vitamins; low kilojoule diet	B2, B3 Increase food intake
	Scaling of skin around nostrils (naso-labial seborrhea)	Inadequate vitamins	B2, B3, B6
Lips	Redness and swelling of mouth or lips (cheilosis)	Inadequate vitamins	B2, B3
	Cracks at side of mouth (andular fissures)	Inadequate B group vitamins, especially B6, B2, B3; iron	B6, B2, B3 Iron

Nails	Spoon-shaped brittle, ridged white spots		Iron Silica and fatty acids Zinc
Gums	Abnormally red and bleeding	Deficient vitamin C	Vitamin C bioflavonoids
Hair	Dull, dry, falls out easily	Low in protein, fatty and amino acids	Fish oil, evening primrose oil, silica
Tongue	Raw, red, cracked, swollen, pale, smooth, slick, magenta	Lack of folic acid, niacin, riboflavin B6, B12, iron	Supplement with these vitamins and minerals
Eyes	Pale eye membranes	Iron deficiency	Iron
	Spots of dryness conjunctivitis, soft or dull cornea	Vitamin A deficiency	Vitamin A
	Redness and fissured eyelids	Vitamin B deficiency	B6, riboflavin niacin
Legs	Edema	Poor protein	Amino acids
Skin	Darkness, roughness, bruising, purple pinhead spots, Lack of rebound, Pressure sores	Vitamin deficiency Dehydration	B3, B12, folic acid, Vitamin A, fatty acids, Vitamin C and K Vitamin C Vitamin C Vitamin C, E, zinc

Dietary inadequacies of schoolchildren in Australia.

The following National dietary survey of schoolchildren (aged 10–15 years) is the result of studies carried out by the Department of Community Services and Health, in 1985.

Retinol Equivalents (Vitamin A)

RDI Boys 12–15 years 725ug/day
Girls 12–15 years 725ug/day

Results showed that 49.6% of boys aged 12 years were receiving less than the recommended dietary intake. 52.6% of girls aged 12 years were receiving less than the recommended dietary intake.

Vitamin B1 (Thiamin)

RDI Boys 12 years of age   1.2mg
Results showed that 44.2% of boys aged 12 years and 37.7% of girls received less than the RDI daily of Vitamin B1.

Vitamin B2 (Riboflavin)

RDI Boys 12 years of age   1.8mg
Results showed that 33.6% of boys and 38.7% of girls received less than the RDI daily of Vitamin B2.

Vitamin B3 (Nicotinic Acid)

RDI 12–15 year old boys   19–21mg
    12–15 year old girls   17–19mg
Results showed that 21.1% of 12 year old boys and 26.9% of 12 year old girls received less than the RDI daily.

Vitamin C (Ascorbic Acid)

RDI 12–15 year old boys   30mg
    12–15 year old girls   30mg
Results showed that 22.0% of 12 year old boys and 17.6% of 12 year old girls received less than the RDI

Iron

RDI 12–15 year old boys   10–13mg
    12–15 year old girls   10–13mg
Results showed that 48.9% of 12 year old boys and 64.8% of 12 year old girls received less than the RDI

Calcium

RDI 12–15 year old boys   1200mg
    12–15 year old girls   1000mg
Results showed that 75.1% of 12 year old boys and 71.4% of 12 year old girls received less than the RDI

Zinc

RDI 12–15 year old boys   12–18mg
     12–15 year old girls   12–18mg
  Results showed that 71.5% of 12 year old boys and 82.0% of 12 year old girls received less than the RDI

Magnesium

RDI 12–15 year old boys   260mg
     12–15 year old girls   240mg
  Results showed that 52% of 12 year old boys and 57.6% of 12 year old girls received less than the RDI
  These results show that we must look to improving the nutritional value of foods for our children. However, based on the evidence above, supplementation could be of benefit.

Supplements:

One Naturetime Multi-Vitamin Mineral Formula tablet daily.
  Increase intake of calcium food, dairy products, or soy milk and fresh fruit, vegetables, lean meat, fish and nuts.

Dietary Inadequacies of Adults in Australia.

The following is a National Dietary Survey of Adults carried out by the Department of Community Services and Health, in 1983.

Retinol Equivalent (Vitamin A)

RDI Men 19–64 years of age   750ug
     Women 19–54 years of age   750ug
  Results showed that 40.9% of men aged 35–44 years and 48.9% of women aged 35–44 received less than the RDI daily.

Vitamin B1 (Thiamin)

RDI Men 19–64 years of age   1.1mg.
     Women 19–54 years of age   0.8mg.
  Results showed that 39.0% of men aged 35–44 years and 39.4% of women aged 35–44 years received less than the RDI daily.

Vitamin B2 (Riboflavin)

RDI Men 25–64 years of age   1.7mg
      Women 25–54 years of age   1.2mg
  Results showed that 35.2% of men aged 35–44 years and 35.3% of women aged 35–44 years received less than the RDI

Vitamin B3 (Nicotinic Acid)

RDI Men 19–64 years of age   18–20mg
      Women 19–54 years of age   12–14mg
  Results showed that 6.6% of men aged 35–44 years and 6.5% of women aged 35–44 years received less than the RDI daily.

Vitamin C (Ascorbic Acid)

RDI Men 19–64 years of age   40mg
      Women 19–54 years of age   30mg
  Results showed that 25.2% of men aged 35–44 years and 24.3% of women aged 35–44 years received less than the RDI daily.

Iron

RDI Men 19–64 years of age   5–7mg
      Women 19–54 years of age   12–16mg
  Results showed that 2.9% of men aged 35–44 years and 75.3% of women aged 35–44 years received less than the RDI daily.

Calcium

RDI Men 19–64 years of age   800mg
      Women 19–54 years of age   800mg
  Results showed that 52.2% of men aged 35–44 years and 66.4% of women aged 35–44 years received less than the RDI daily.

Zinc

RDI Men 19–64 years of age   12–16mg
      Women 19–54 years of age   12–16mg
  Results showed that 52.9% of men aged 35–44 years and 83.4% of women aged 35–44 years received less than the RDI daily.

Magnesium

RDI Men 19–64 years of age   320mg
     Women 19–54 years of age   270mg
   Results showed that 35% of men aged 35–44 years and 55.7%
of women aged 35–44 years received less than the RDI daily.

Supplements

One Naturetime Multi-Vitamin Mineral Formula tablet daily.
   Increase intake of calcium food, dairy products, or soy milk and
fresh fruit, vegetables, lean meat, fish and nuts.

PART II
THE A–Z OF COMMON ILLNESSES

i. Supplements are available from your health food store and pharmacy.

ii. There is a comprehensive guide to all herbs mentioned, in PART III of this book: Guide to Herbs Used in this Book.

ACNE OR ACNE VULGARIS

Up to 80% of Australian teenagers are affected by acne. Those who suffer the most are those with an oily skin. The main cause of acne in adolescents is the increased production of hormones: oestrogen in the young woman and androgen in the youth. This increase in hormones stimulates the sebaceous glands of the skin, producing an oversupply of sebum and it is this oily substance that normally keeps the skin healthy. With clogging of the pores blackheads and whiteheads appear, which can become inflamed causing common acne.

Diet is extremely important and oily foods such as nuts, dairy products, chocolates and junk foods should definitely be avoided. Soy milk should be considered instead of milk. Plenty of exercise and the importance of cleansing the skin cannot be over-emphasised, especially with soaps designed to keep the skin in a healthy state. Exfoliation is also necessary and a scrub should be used to remove the dead layers of skin which will open the pores to allow the sebum to escape without clogging. The pimples should be treated with a gel containing tea-tree oil. Tea-tree oil is an excellent anti-bacterial product which will not damage the skin.

Removal of blackheads should not be attempted unless the area has been sufficiently softened with special lotions to enable their easy extraction without damaging the skin.

If a program is followed, even though acne itself cannot be

completely prevented, scarring can be kept to a minimum and quite often the amount of acne present is not of concern. Always remember that acne can cause severe psychological problems, especially in young teenage girls, and if you are giving advice then be tactful.

Hair care is also extremely important. Regular washing and care of the hair can also help reduce the oily skin condition.

Foods that are very high in Vitamin A have shown good results with acne sufferers and with most skin conditions, food containing zinc should also be considered. Owing to the poor quality of foods and eating habits of teenagers, supplementation could be of benefit under these circumstances.

SUPPLEMENTS

vitamin A	up to 100,000 IU daily for 4 weeks, then stop for a fortnight

Note: vitamin A can be toxic if taken in large amounts. See your practitioner before starting large amounts.

zinc (elemental)	25 mg per day
Efamol Marine (evening primrose oil and marine lipids)	2 three times a day:
vitamin E (tocopheryl succinate)	400 IU twice daily

avoid inorganic iron (inactivates vitamin E)
avoid female hormones (antagonistic to vitamin E)

vitamin C	2000 mg daily
Echinacea complex	one tablet 3 times daily

External treatment

tea-tree gel	once daily
anti-bacterial face wash (based on tea-tree oil)	once daily

AGEING SPOTS

Ageing spots are little brown spots that often first appear on the back of the hands. Ageing spots do not indicate disease. They may be unsightly but are not a problem. Most people develop them as they get older. We can prevent the occurrence of these spots. This condition is also known as amyloidosis. What we can do is take antioxidants. We should include foods in our diet that are rich in Vitamins A, C and E. Because they are so important in the prevention of many ailments, antioxidants are discussed in this book several times. They prevent free radicals in the body from damaging our cells and causing premature ageing. Part of this cell damage may be these ageing spots which appear on the back of your hands.

If you feel your diet is lacking then supplement it with a formula which contains the antioxidant vitamins A, C and E, plus zinc and the herb ginseng. This type of formula can help prevent many age-related problems. Cataracts can also be prevented by taking antioxidants. These findings were reported in the Proceedings of the National Academy of Sciences, July 1979 and 'Photochemistry and Photobiology', 36, 6, 1982.) However, ageing spots are probably the first sign of antioxidant deficiency in the diet. If you take the antioxidants early in life, then the chances are you won't develop ageing spots or they will be reduced in number.

Keep up the good eating habits, live a good healthy lifestyle and supplement your diet with antioxidants.

For more information see Antioxidants.

Supplements

cod liver oil
(contains vitamin A, D and essential fatty acids)   5 ml daily

beta-carotene (natural)   3000 mcg three times daily

vitamin C
(ascorbic acid)   2000 mg daily or more

vitamin E   300 IU daily

selenium   50 mcg daily (prescribed by medical practitioner)

garlic   include in food

Korean ginseng   75 mg per day

Bio Zinc
(contains 25 mg of elemental zinc)   one tablet daily

AIDS (see Immune System)

ALCOHOL

Alcohol consumption is of growing concern in our community. Alcohol can both directly and indirectly cause many illnesses and associated nutritional deficiencies. Experimental studies have shown that 81% of chronic alcoholics treated with a well-balanced diet plus supplements were still sober after six months. Only 38% of alcoholics were still sober after six months when treated with a standard hospital diet (as reported by R. Guenther in the *International Journal of Biosocial Research in 1983*).

It is important if one is a heavy drinker to reduce or stop alcohol consumption and supplement a well balanced diet with a multi-vitamin mineral formula. Extra water needs to be consumed as well, alcohol causes dehydration of the brain which may also result in brain damage.

The liver processes alcohol and the heavy drinker runs the risk of liver damage and cirrhosis of the liver. This disease is dangerous and if not treated properly and alcohol consumption stopped can be fatal. Experimental studies have shown that vitamin C may reduce the effects of alcohol toxicity. Other studies have shown that vitamin C is usually deficient in alcohol related diseases and when taken before or during alcohol ingestion may help prevent alcohol-induced fatty liver, fatty liver precedes cirrhosis.

The herb milk thistle has also been shown to help prevent and reverse certain types of liver damage caused by alcohol ingestion. (For more information see Liver Health)

SUPPLEMENTS

Milk thistle	1 ml of 1:1 fluid extract 3 times daily
Naturetime B+C	one tablet twice daily
Naturetime multi-vitamin mineral	one tablet daily
water	6 to 8 glasses per day

ALLERGIES

Sometimes people have allergies to certain foods they eat and this can cause a number of different symptoms ranging from indigestion and irritable bowel syndrome to asthma and dermatitis. There are a number of tests that can be used to find what foods cause an adverse reaction.

Migraine headaches can follow the consumption of hard cheese, chocolate or oranges. Migraine headaches can be reduced by 90% if diet is observed. Eliminate these foods and watch the result.

There are tests to determine food allergies. A cytotoxic blood test compares the reaction of the blood to as many as 120 different types of foods and can help in the formulation of a diet that will assist the patient back to good health. A RAST (Radio-Allergo Sorbent Test) allergy test is also useful.

Seek expert advice if you believe you react adversely to certain foods in your diet.

The following balancing diet can also help you determine the foods that are causing many allergic reactions.

BALANCING DIET
(Elimination Diet)

This diet is to balance the pH of the body (acidity and alkalinity) and at the same time, by the way of reactive and non-reactive foods, bring the body into harmony.

The following is a list of foods that you can eat in the first stage of the diet. Steam your food slowly, do not overcook it.

*herbal teas — peppermint, spearmint

*carrots, celery, lettuce

*potatoes should be eaten at each meal. (Don't use new potatoes or potatoes with any green spots as these contain solanine which is poisonous.) Use white rice if you are allergic to potatoes.

*bananas, pears

*olive oil

*small servings of scaled fish

DAY 1

Bake 10 potatoes. Steam 8 carrots and when tender add the baked potatoes. Use a little olive oil and mash.

BREAKFAST: Before eating, chew 2 slippery elm tablets.

Eat a serving of the carrots and baked potatoes with herbal tea.

MORNING TEA: Peppermint tea and a piece of fruit.

LUNCH: Chew one slippery elm before and one after lunch. Some of the carrots and potatoes with boiled greens and herbal tea,

or

potato sandwich with unleavened Lebanese or pita bread if you can't cook lunch, with herbal tea

DINNER: Chew one slippery elm before and one after dinner.

steamed fish (small serve) with potatoes and greens and herbal tea.

Continue this diet for 5 days.

DAY 6

The following foods may be added to the diet but not fried:

farm fresh eggs

honey

butter

whole-grain bread.

Continue with this diet for the next 5 days.

DAY 12

You can now add your normal foods such as grilled chicken, steamed fish and vegetables. Add other natural foods to the diet. This must be done by adding one food at a time (see alkaline foods). If, when a food is added, an allergic reaction is noted, then remove that food from your diet for a minimum of three months before trying it again. By the end of the third week you will have compiled a list of foods that agree with you and do not cause any allergic reactions.

This diet should be beneficial if used once per month.

Your water supply, along with artificial food ingredients, could be the source of the toxic pollutants in your body.

SUPPLEMENTS

vitamin B6	25 mg daily — this can help reduce monosodium glutamate sensitivity.
vitamin C + bioflavonoids	1000 mg morning and night — this lowers elevated blood histamine levels
natural vitamin E	500 IU daily — anti histamine properties
evening primrose oil	1 capsule 3 times daily
Ephedra	800 mg 3 times daily — used for hay fever and hives (urticaria)

Note: *Ephedra* contains ephedrine and should not be used if suffering hypertension.

ALZHEIMER'S DISEASE (see Memory)

ANALGESICS

Natural Pain Relief

Many people are rightly concerned about using manufactured 'pain-killers' as these may cause side effects. However, there are some herbs that contain quite strong analgesic properties. White willow bark contains constituents very similar to aspirin. It was in looking at what the ancient apothecaries did with this herb that we were able to develop aspirin.

White willow bark does not produce the side effects of the other analgesics so it can be very gentle in its pain-relieving properties. It is effective for headache, muscular ache and backache. It is available in health food stores. The herb is usually mixed with other herbs that also have slight analgesic properties.

It has been shown in experimental studies that D L phenylalanine can relieve pain when patients are taken off other medications. The study noted over 50% reduction in pain. If pain continues for a long time then you should see your practitioner.

SUPPLEMENTS

Esprin   contains white willow bark 2700 mg
devil's claw 200 mg
magnesium phosphate 100 mg

Use Esprin as you would aspirin for temporary relief of pain.

betony   1000 mg 3 times daily — for headache
associated with nervous tension

D L–phenylalanine   250 mg 3 times daily
(amino acid)

ANTIOXIDANTS

Antioxidants can prevent free radicals damaging your cells. These free radicals are a by-product of the metabolism of oxygen. The same radicals cause an apple to go brown when cut and exposed to the air, or butter to become rancid. Commonsense tells us that if our cells are damaged it will show in the form of premature ageing and reduced resistance to infection. Antioxidants, such as vitamins A, C and E, in correct dosages provide the tools to remove the impurities. This allows the cell membrane to be properly protected, hence ensuring that the cell lives its full, normal life.

The main antioxidants are beta-carotene, vitamin C, vitamin E, certain amino acids such as DL-methionine, zinc and B6. Certain trace elements such as selenium, which is found in garlic, is also a very important antioxidant. Much scientific research has now been carried out into the use of antioxidants such as A, C and E to show whether or not they can prevent premature ageing or slow down the ageing process in animals. The results of these tests have been promising and in animal experiments, the length of life has been increased.

These studies also showed that ageing spots or amyloidosis can be decreased with the use of antioxidants. Professor Linus Pauling, the twice Nobel Prize recipient and Professor of Chemistry at Stanford University in the USA, has suggested that we all should be taking antioxidants to help combat the pollutants, poisons and toxins that exist in our atmosphere, our water and our foods. He believes that if we do take antioxidants, it is possible to add twenty-five years to our life.

Further evidence is given when Dr Mark Florence, Senior Research Scientist for the CSIRO, states, 'I have studied the effect of anti-oxidants for 10 years and there are good biochemical reasons why they should work.' He also stated, 'I would confidently advise people to take them.'

Researchers at the University of Western Ontario, Toronto, have also found antioxidants such as vitamin E and vitamin C in large doses could help prevent cataracts (the clouding of the eye lens) in old age.

I am sure that, with the agreement of eminent people such as Dr Florence, Dr Linus Pauling and many other researchers, antioxidants do work. It is possible to increase our quality of life and build the immune system to a level where we can help combat many of the normal viral cold, flu and other ailments that plague our everyday lives.

I confidently recommend a formula containing beta-carotene, vitamin C, vitamin E, vitamins B1, B5, B6, methionine and zinc. There is ample evidence to show that these, in combination, are the best form for an antioxidant preparation. The addition of garlic would be an extremely good idea because of its trace elements, anti blood-clotting and cholesterol-lowering properties. The ancient Chinese herb, ginseng has the ability to improve or increase physical and mental capacity and improve resistance to viral infection.

What we are looking for is a formula which lengthens lives and improves the quality of life.

SUPPLEMENT

The Bio ACE antioxidant formula contains:
beta-carotene
vitamin E
vitamin C
garlic
ginseng
zinc
vitamins B1, B5, B6

Take 1 tablet up to 3 times daily.

ARTHRITIS (also see Gout)

Arthritis is a debilitating disease which affects many Australians, including children. There are many types of arthritis. Rheumatoid arthritis, gout and osteoarthritis are the main forms.

Rheumatoid arthritis

Rheumatoid arthritis is a chronic painful disease that can affect all joints in the body, the hands, wrists, ankles, toes, neck and hips. Rheumatoid arthritis is thought to be an auto immune disease, one in which the body produces a disordered immunological response which can cause injury to normal parts of the body.

Major psychological or physical factors in life can trigger rheumatoid arthritis. Some of the first symptoms may be weight loss, pains in the joints (especially in the morning) and hot and swollen joints.

Each attack seems to be a little worse than the last. Eventually there is deformity in the joints following loss of minerals, adhesion of the tissues to the bone and limpy nodules around the affected area.

To help alleviate the pain and reduce the discomfort, we must look at our diet first (see Diet for crystal arthritis) Avoid foods such as tomatoes and oranges which have been known to cause problems. Also increase your intake of vegetables and fruit and reduce the intake of red meats and acid foods. Some nuts and even wheat can be a problem. Look towards rice, rye and buckwheat. Plenty of fresh water is essential: 6 to 8 glasses a day. All of this can make a difference.

It is a good idea to supplement the diet with cod liver oil or fish oil as recent research has shown that fish oil can help relieve the pain of arthritis. These supplements contain essential fatty acids that have anti-inflammatory properties. Celery seed can also help. Buy this from the health food store. It is present in a celery complex. This complex should also contain the herbs *Apium* and *Guaiacum*. All these herbs have properties that can help relieve inflammation and detoxify the joints.

For the pain of arthritis the herbs white willow bark and devil's claw taken in combination are very effective. White willow bark has similar properties to aspirin.

You should exercise daily but don't overdo it. Swimming and walking are good.

SUPPLEMENTS

evening primrose oil   2 capsules 3 times daily
fish oil 1000   1 capsule 3 times daily

vitamin C	2000 mg daily
pantothenic acid (Vitamin B5)	200 mg daily
multivitamin/mineral	1 daily
white willow bark	2700 mg twice daily (found in herbal analgesic formula)
celery seeds	400 mg twice daily
devils claw	200 mg twice daily
Guaiacum	400 mg twice daily
calcium fluoride 3 X	3 times daily
silica	25 mg twice daily
calcium phosphate	(up to 1000 mg of elemental calcium daily

ASTHMA

More people suffer from asthma these days than 20 years ago. Pollution plays a large part in precipitating asthma attacks among many sensitive people. As well we tend to add artificial colourings, flavourings and preservatives to our foods and these exacerbate allergies and asthma in sensitive people. Avoid foods containing additives (see Allergies). People have allergies to other foods and a cytotoxic blood test may be carried out to determine what other foods should be avoided. Dairy products are one of the most common as these are mucus-forming and should not be included in the asthmatic diet. Use soybean milk. A RAST test is also helpful in determining other allergies.

Supplementing the diet with cod liver oil can also be beneficial as it contains essential fatty acids that have anti-inflammatory effects. Vitamin A can help strengthen the mucus membranes.

Herbs such as *Euphorbia, Grindelia* and thyme are valuable and can usually be found in complex form at your health food store or pharmacy. These herbs prevent asthma attacks and bronchial spasms. This makes breathing easier.

It is important to stay on the medication prescribed by your general practitioner. However, if you make these dietary changes and supplement your diet with cod liver oil and *Euphorbia* you may not need stronger medication.

SUPPLEMENTS

cod liver oil	take 5 ml (one teaspoon) daily
evening primrose oil	take two capsules morning and night
Euphorbia	these herbs are usually found in
Grindelia	combination from your health food
Senega	store or pharmacy. Follow directions
Thyme	on bottle. For a stronger formula, see
	your naturopath.
Glycyrrhiza	steroid-like activity

ATHLETES AND REGULAR EXERCISERS

Do athletes, joggers, regular exercisers and people who do heavy physical work require special treatment?

They may be at risk because they have low levels of essential nutrients in their bodies.

A study carried out by the Department of Sport has shown that our athletes are running the risk of having a low serum (blood) concentration of certain nutrients. This has been backed up by further experiments to show that certain micro-nutrients such as vitamin E and other antioxidant vitamins can be utilised at a faster rate by those who are striving and taking part in endurance athletic activity. Athletes need to look at eating a well-balanced diet and supplements because they are pushing their bodies beyond the normal limit.

Heavy workouts build up lactic acid in the muscles which produces free radicals. These can cause cell damage so it is important for athletes to take extra antioxidants if they are working out or training hard.

Dr Lester Packer of the University of California at Berkeley, has shown that free radicals damage muscle cells. He found evidence of damage to all major membranes of muscle tissue caused by free radicals following athletic activity. He suggested an antioxidant formula containing beta-carotene, vitamin E and vitamin C to help prevent this damage.

If you are an athlete striving to achieve higher levels of fitness and performance in your athletic field, then consider supplementing with a Bio ACE type formula containing A, C and E, the antioxidant vitamins. However there is no substitute for a good well-balanced diet.

Consider a little extra protein if you are engaging in heavy, muscle-ripping exercises. Amino acids, found in protein, are the building blocks of life needed to repair muscle tissue damaged during heavy exercise. There are 8 essential amino acids which must be obtained from your diet. Eggs and dairy products are the best sources. Use egg whites and skim milk as these will not increase cholesterol.

Supplements of the minerals magnesium, potassium and zinc is helpful, especially if you experience cramps or muscle pain after exercise.

SUPPLEMENTS

Bio ACE antioxidant formula containing vitamins A, C, E and K	one 3 times daily
zinc (elemental)	25 mg daily
vitamin E	500 IU daily
selenium (trace element)	found in garlic and eggs
garlic	2000 mg (fresh herb equivalent) daily

Skim milk and egg whites are excellent sources of amino acids.
Make a milk shake:
Ingredients 2 egg whites
1 teaspoon black strap molasses
1 teaspoon honey
1 banana
½ teaspoon yeast
2 glasses of skim or low fat milk
Blend and drink.

This is a high protein drink that also contains all essential vitamins and minerals. It is ideal for body builders.

BABIES' PROBLEMS

Colic

Wind is a real problem and causes much discomfort in babies. A baby's smile is often caused by wind. Blueness around the mouth can be a sign of wind.

The size of the hole in the teat of a bottle needs to be right. If it is too large or small your baby will suck and swallow air. This wind builds up in the stomach and causes pain.

Most mothers experiment and find the best way to burp baby but sometimes there is still a problem.

A little peppermint tea will help expel the wind and settle baby's stomach. Dill tea is also recommended.

SUPPLEMENT

peppermint tea   10 to 20 ml up to three times a day
   or dill tea   or when required for wind

Nappy rash

One of the many problems suffered by babies is nappy rash. Teething or a wet nappy can cause a rash which can be very irritating. Babies cry with pain. Powders made up at home can be helpful. One of them is cornflour and zinc oxide. You can buy these ingredients from your chemist and mix them together. It is an old remedy and is very soothing.

Another thing you can use is apricot kernel oil mixed with vitamin E, or an apricot E oil. When applied to the rash it can ease the irritation.

Nappy rash can also be caused by a problem with the diet. Sometimes thrush or *Candida albicans* can cause it and if that is the case, *Lactobacillus acidophilus* can be of benefit. *Lactobacillus acidophilus* can be found in natural yoghurts. Also, if it is a *Candida albicans* problem (thrush), a little tea-tree oil applied to the area can help kill the infection but it must be diluted and is best diluted in glycerine.

SUPPLEMENTS

one third tea-tree oil and two-thirds glycerine, applied externally with a cotton bud.

multivitamins for children as directed (crush and put in food).

BACK PAIN

We must look after our backs. Back pain or injury can be caused by just picking up a tissue. We must remember that the head weighs about 7 kilograms and this puts a tremendous strain on the lower back when bending over and not bending the knees. It is very important to lift things correctly. Squatting down is always the answer no matter what you are picking up. It is also important to hold the object being lifted and carried close to the body.

Back injuries and back pain contribute to massive absenteeism in the Australian workforce. Back damage can be caused from gardening, normal household duties or heavy lifting. The pain can be excruciating and can affect our everyday life. Back pain can be caused by strained muscles, damage to one or more of the discs, and pressure on a nerve.

If you have back pain there are many things that can help. Taking analgesics only masks the symptoms and relieves the pain but does not solve the problem. Prevention is better than cure. If the back problem is muscular then the herb valerian can help relax the muscles and reduce the pain. A celery complex containing celery seeds, an anti-rheumatic herb, and *Guaiacum*, a herb that has anti-inflammatory and anti-rheumatic qualities, are very beneficial. These herbs help reduce inflammation and acid build-up in the area, quickly helping the return of movement without pain.

Salves containing wintergreen oil can help during the acute stage as well as a supplement with white willow bark. (This has similar properties to aspirin as mentioned previously under Analgesics.)

SUPPLEMENTS

A celery complex containing celery seeds and *Guaiacum*	one 3 times daily
iron phosphate	15 mg three times daily
valerian (to relax muscles)	300 mg twice daily with food
silica	25 mg twice daily

For temporary relief of pain take a herbal analgesic which contains

white willow bark	2700 mg every 6 hours or as required
devil's claw	200 mg every 6 hours or as required

Note: See your general practitioner if the pain continues.

BAD BREATH

Halitosis

Finding what causes bad breath is the best way to treat the problem. Certain types of catarrhal problems and lung problems can cause bad breath. These could be sinusitis, emphysema or bronchitis. However, in many cases, the problem of bad breath comes from either teeth or the digestive system.

Proper brushing of the teeth is very important and this will remove rotting food particles that can cause bad breath. Herbs can also help bad breath. One of the most common is parsley. Chlorophyll can also assist.

If our digestive system is causing the problem there are other steps we need to take. It may be that our digestive bacteria is out of balance as there is not enough *Lactobacillus acidophilus* present because of an infestation of *Candida albicans*. This can lead to bad breath, flatulence and indigestion. *Lactobacillus acidophilus* is the bacteria used to make yoghurt and that bacteria lives in the gastro-intestinal tract. It is important for normal digestion so eating plenty of yoghurt each day can help.

As *Lactobacillus acidophilus* can also be reduced following antibiotic therapy or when you suffer from gastroenteritis, a supplement of *Lactobacillus acidophilus* is the best way to normalise the gut flora and lead to good health.

Following all of the above suggestions, drinking plenty of water and having a balanced diet should eliminate the problem.

SUPPLEMENTS

Lactobacillus acidophilus (also found in yoghurt)	once daily
Digestive Aid (contains slippery elm plus plant enzymes)	one tablet 3 times daily
chlorophyll	
peppermint oil	1 or 2 drops twice daily
peppermint tea	4 cups daily

BEDSORES

Bedsores may be caused from the pressure of lying in one part of the body for too long thus reducing the blood supply to the area.

Dead tissue and an ulcer can result. It is important that all body parts must be moved if there is bed confinement each day. This will help maintain good circulation and ensure the normal blood flow containing oxygen and nutrients reaches all parts of the body. Tight clothing can restrict the flow of blood to limbs. Taking vitamin E can help lower the viscosity, or thickness, of the blood improving supply to legs and arms. Vitamin E also has excellent healing properties. Zinc and vitamin C are also important nutrients to include in the diet. Vitamin C and Bio Zinc are needed to help form collagen (the cement of skin) needed for the formation of new tissue and to speed up the healing process.

An ointment that contains comfrey has cell-proliferant properties. It has been used for centuries in healing preparations and was commonly called 'knitbone'. The cream should also contain vitamin E and vitamin A, as these vitamins help speed up the healing process.

SUPPLEMENTS

Bio C	1000 mg
Zinc	25 mg daily
vitamin E	500 IU daily
cod liver oil	5 ml daily

External treatment — use a healing cream containing comfrey, natural vitamin E and A, apricot kernel oil, allantoin

BITES AND STINGS

Bites and stings can be very painful and some people have life-threatening allergic reactions to the venom.

There are many preparations available, manufactured and natural. Our grandmothers used to apply blue-bag to bee stings. There are many other things you can do to help reduce the pain of bites and stings. Bull ant sting can be relieved quite quickly by using the root of the bracken fern. Just pull the fern out, break the root and apply the sap directly to the sting area. It makes a difference.

Sandflies

Taking a B group vitamin in the diet can help prevent sandfly bites. Many people are very allergic to sandfly bites and B group vitamins can help and must be taken before entering an area where there are sandflies.

Box Jellyfish

In Australian waters there are many varieties of jellyfish, in Queensland. The box jellyfish is very dangerous. Its sting can be fatal. Common household vinegar can be very helpful, especially for a box jellyfish bite. It should be applied freely to the area. The tentacles must be removed with tweezers. If the sting is from a box jellyfish send for medical aid.

Bluebottle

With the bluebottle, remove tentacles with tweezers or fingers, wash with water. Apply crushed ice wrapped in a tea towel to the area stung until pain is relieved. If a large area is stung or the casualty is distressed in any way, seek medical aid.

Snake Bite

Australia has many venomous snakes. The taipan, tiger and brown snake are all very poisonous. Others such as the carpet snake and green tree snake are non-venomous.

It is important to leave snakes alone. Many are not aggressive, unless disturbed, and will not usually bite.

If you are bitten and are not absolutely sure that the snake is non-venomous then the following steps need to be taken.

1 The victim must rest. Reassure the person. Don't panic as there is an anti-venom available for all Australian snakes.

2 Apply an elastic bandage starting at the bitten area and around the whole limb. If a person is bitten on the foot then start the bandage around the foot and then continue until the whole leg is covered.

3 Take the casualty to hospital or ring or send for medical aid.

Funnel-web Spider

The Australian funnel-web spider is very poisonous. It is a large black or reddish-brown spider and is found in rock crevices and under logs and rocks along the New South Wales coast and south-east Queensland. The bite is very painful.

The treatment is the same as for snake bite.

Red-back Spider

The red-back spider is common in Australia and lives in old tins, under wood heaps and in dark corners of the house. The red-back has a large red stripe on its back and is a much smaller spider than the funnel web. The bite of a red-back is like a sharp sting and there will be swelling around the bite. The bitten person usually starts to sweat and may become nauseous.

1 Rest the bitten casualty and reassure him/her.
2 Apply ice wrapped in a towel or cold packs to the bitten area. DO NOT BANDAGE. Send for medical aid or take the person to hospital.

Mosquito Bites

Mosquitoes can be very annoying and the best way to treat their bites is to prevent them.

If out in the bush, burning dry cow manure will help keep them away. The odour is not offensive. Citronella or tea-tree oil rubbed on the skin will also keep them away. Be careful not to get oil in your eyes.

If bitten by a mosquito apply bicarbonate of soda or tea-tree oil to the affected area and the itch will soon be relieved.

SUPPLEMENTS

B group vitamins   1 tablet morning and night

Also see Allergies.

BLOOD PRESSURE (also see Hawthorn)

High blood pressure is a very dangerous condition and if you are under a doctor's supervision for this problem then you must advise him or her of any changes you wish to make to your diet.

Vitamin E can help lower blood pressure. Drs Shute and Shute were pioneers in the use of vitamin E in the treatment of heart disease. Vitamin E's action on the cardiovascular system (under supervision) should not be overlooked. Vitamin E can also help prevent blood clots forming in the blood. This and its ability to lower blood viscosity makes vitamin E important for the treatment of many circulatory disorders (see Hawthorn Berry).

Herbs such as hawthorn and garlic have been shown to have a favourable effect on the cardiovascular system. Hawthorn improves coronary blood flow and causes peripheral vasodilation. This action reduces the myocardium's (heart muscle) need for oxygen and also lowers blood pressure.

Garlic has a direct effect on the heart muscle and has mild vasodilating properties. It too can lower blood pressure. Garlic and hawthorn help lower blood cholesterol levels and can help reverse arteriosclerosis (hardening of the arteries). These herbs, in combination, are very beneficial and useful when used for the prevention and/or treatment of high blood pressure.

Medical trials have shown that evening primrose oil can also help to lower blood pressure and cholesterol. It therefore should be included in the diet if high blood pressure is a problem.

Salt, as we all should know by now, can cause high blood pressure in some people. Salt, taken to excess, causes problems in the retention of fluid. This excess fluid is caused by the need to dissolve the excess sodium and hold it in solution. This causes an increase in the blood volume and a corresponding rise in blood pressure. This increase in blood pressure places a larger working load on the heart and circulatory system.

The average Australian, according to the Australian Heart Foundation, only requires 200 mg of sodium per day to maintain a healthy working life. We do not need to add sodium chloride (salt) to our food as most tinned or packaged foods contain added salt. There are a number of good publications that list the salt contained in many foods and it would be a good idea to get a copy of the *Nutritional Almanac*.

The average Australian consumes between 1 and 3 teaspoons of table salt per day giving them an average of 400 mg of sodium and this level is far too high.

I recall the case of a woman patient who, although taking her doctor's medication, still had problems in keeping her blood pressure under control. On analysing her diet we found that she had a salt intake of around 7000 mg per day. I placed her on a low salt diet in combination with a herbal preparation containing hawthorn and garlic. This medication reduced her blood pressure to 120/80 (normal). Soon after she was able to completely stop taking the prescribed drugs (this was done with her doctor's permission).

Note if you have high blood pressure, you should see your general practitioner as soon as possible.

SUPPLEMENTS

evening primrose oil	2 capsules 3 times daily
hawthorn	500 mg dried herb twice daily
garlic	500 mg dried herb twice daily
lime flower	750 mg dried herb twice daily
vitamin E	start with low dose and increase to 500 IU daily.

Also see Heart Disease.

BOWEL POLYPS

Bowel polyps (polyposis) are benign growths which develop on the colon wall. They are mainly familial, and if not attended to may form an adenoma and become cancerous. The medical treatment for polyps is surgery either by removal of the polyps or by removal of the bowel.

There is a lot which can be done to both prevent and eliminate bowel polyps. Diet is very important. The diet must be high in fibre and low in animal fat. Vegetables containing beta-carotene can prevent polyps becoming cancerous.

Dr Jerome DeCosse of Wisconsin's Department of Surgery and Pathology, discovered that vitamin C reduced the number of, or eliminated, bowel polyps in 8 out of 10 patients.

SUPPLEMENTS

vitamin C	5000-10000 mg daily
beta-carotene (natural)	6 mg daily with main meal
Bio ACE antioxidant formula	1 tablet twice daily

BRAN

Many people are confused by the information they receive about brans — wheat bran, rice bran, oat bran. The bran is part of the whole kernel of wheat, rice or oats. It is the part underneath the outer layer of husk. Bran products are made by removing the husk of the kernel and the abrasive milling of the thin bran layers.

Some bran products such as rice bran also include the germ, making them highly nutritious as the germ is rich in many vitamins, minerals and essential fatty acids.

Bran contains two types of dietary fibre, soluble and insoluble. It is the insoluble fibre that helps the body by providing bulky fibre and promoting bowel regularity. Wheat bran contains around 33.3% insoluble fibre, rice bran 23% and oat bran around 5.5%.

If regularity is the problem, then it may be that the diet is lacking in insoluble fibre. If this is the case, then including 60 grams of rice or wheat bran will help. Drink 6 to 8 glasses of water daily as water moves food through the digestive tract.

The soluble fibre found in bran is as important as the insoluble fibre. Soluble fibre can help reduce the risk of certain types of heart disease by reducing blood cholesterol levels and improving the HDL:LDL ratio. HDL, or high density lipoproteins are responsible for carrying excess cholesterol from the blood stream back to the liver. The liver uses cholesterol to manufacture bile salts which are needed to emulsify fats in the intestine for absorption. LDL, or low density lipoprotein, transports cholesterol to different parts of the body for use by the cells. However, excess LDLs are deposited on the artery walls if not used. This can lead to a hardening and narrowing of these blood vessels resulting in cardiovascular disease.

Oat bran contains the highest percentage of soluble fibre at 4.8%, followed by rice bran at 2.5% and wheat bran at 2.0%. The latest technical information shows that rice bran and oat bran are equal in their ability to lower total blood cholesterol levels.

Rice bran has five times the insoluble dietary fibre of oat bran and more soluble fibre than wheat bran. It can help maintain a healthy colon and promote regularity, as well as caring for the cardiovascular system by helping lower cholesterol.

Psyllium is a natural grain and the husks make an excellent fibre, helping lower cholesterol and maintaining regularity. Psyllium was recently reported in the Archives of Internal Medicine 148, 292, 1988, which stated that psyllium, by removing bile acid from the intestine and preventing their reabsorption, lowered blood cholesterol levels. This action is the result of the use by the body of cholesterol in the manufacture of more bile salts.

SUPPLEMENTS

Psyllium husks   2 teaspoons in orange juice morning and night.

BRONCHITIS

(Acute) Bronchitis is inflammation of the bronchial tubes caused by either bacterial or viral infections. The symptoms usually start with a head cold, slight fever and associated muscle ache which may radiate to the back. There is a cough which is unproductive at first and happens mainly at night. This is shortly followed by the appearance of yellowish phlegm, a hacking cough and higher fever.

The fever can be controlled using white willow bark (see 'Analgesics'). It is also important to use a vaporiser at night, as this helps to lessen the cough and loosen the phlegm. A mixture of winter green oil, camphor, menthol and eucalyptus mixed in equal parts and added to the vaporiser will make breathing easier. Do not go into cold air after using the vaporiser.

There are a number of herbs to loosen mucus build-up and soothe inflamed mucous membranes. They include mullein, horehound and pleurisy root, liquorice root and *Euphorbia*. These herbs taken in combination will help relieve the symptoms. Vitamin C, garlic and *Echinacea* will help control the infection.

A good way to take garlic is take a baked potato, place a clove of garlic in the centre with a little olive oil, mash the potato and eat it hot. It may make you smell of garlic but the aroma of the garlic helps clear the nose and fights the infection in the lungs.

SUPPLEMENTS

vitamin C	1000 mg twice daily
cod liver oil	5 ml daily
mullein	1500 mg twice daily obtained from your practitioner
horehound	1000 mg twice daily obtained from your practitioner
pleurisy root	500 mg twice daily obtained from your practitioner
liquorice root (*Glycyrriza*)	500 mg twice daily
liquorice complex	1 tablet 3 times daily
Echinacea	400 mg twice daily
garlic	2000 mg fresh herb or equivalent daily

iron phosphate   17 mg 3 times daily
potassium chloride   32 mg 3 times daily

These minerals can be found in combination in a cold tablet formula.

BRUISING OR BRUISES

Women seem to bruise more easily than men. Bumping an area can lead to bleeding underneath the skin. This bleeding spreads and the blood is seen through the skin as a blue or black bruise.

Bruising can be the result of dietary deficiencies. Vitamin C is very important, along with the bioflavonoids. These are required by the body to help maintain capillary strength. If you lack vitamin C and bioflavonoids in your diet then bruising and star capillaries will appear. Your diet should be rich in fresh leafy green vegetables and fruit as they contain all of these important nutrients. However, if your diet is lacking, then supplement the diet with vitamin C and bioflavonoids. These substances are extremely important.

There are also other causes of bruising and/or bleeding. Haemophilia and leukaemia are rare diseases than can result in unusual persistent bruising. These conditions must be referred to your doctor.

SUPPLEMENTS

bioflavonoids and   2000 mg daily
  vitamin C

vitamin E (natural)   500 IU daily

zinc (Bio-Zinc)   1 daily (contains 25 mg zinc)

External treatment   rub on area twice daily to bring
comfrey ointment   out bruising and speed the healing
                            process

BURNS

There are two types of burns. Deep-thickness burns which affect the whole skin and deeper tissue and the skin may look black and charred or white. As the nerve endings are often damaged there may be no pain. Superficial burns occur on the surface layers of the skin. They are usually red and may have blisters. Burns can be caused by steam, boiling water, fire, chemicals, sun and friction. As burns can lead to serious infection you need to see your doctor.

Immediately after a burn pour cold water on the burn, or apply an ice pack. This will help stop the burn from spreading, and reduce the pain. (Running water is best and should be run over the burnt area for at least 10 minutes.)

If the burn is not serious it still can be painful and left untreated, can lead to infection and scarring. You need to heal burns quickly. There are many things that can be done to hasten the healing process.

The herb *Aloe vera* is of great benefit for treating burns. The plant can be peeled back and the gel taken and rubbed on the burn. This will really speed up healing and help relieve the pain. *Aloe vera* gel can be bought from a health food store or pharmacy.

As new skin forms following a burn, there is a need for extra Vitamin C and zinc in the diet. Vitamin C forms the cement or the collagen of skin. These and Aloe vera gel will heal the burn very quickly. Vitamin E, taken as a supplement and applied to the area after the initial treatment will help prevent scarring.

If a burn is full-thickness or covering a large area of the body it may require emergency medical treatment. In this case only use cold water on the burn before seeking treatment, and cover the area with a sterile burns' dressing.

SUPPLEMENTS

vitamin E	500 IU daily
Bio-zinc	1 tablet daily
vitamin C + bioflavonoids	2000 mg daily

External treatment
Aloe vera gel
vitamin E cream

CALCIUM

It is now known that 70% of Australian women do not get enough calcium in their diets (according to recommended dietary intake of the National Health and Research Council). This is particularly prevalent after menopause when many women show a sharp drop in calcium intake. Due to a decrease in vitamin and mineral content in our foods over the past few years and the leaching of very important minerals from our soils, we are in the predicament where we could really be called a mineral starved society.

Tests carried out by the American Department of Agriculture in 1984 involving some 1000 crops showed that calcium levels over a 4-year period decreased by as much as 41%. This points to the need for a supplement containing a natural form of calcium in order to bring our dietary calcium level up to that recommended by the National Health and Research Council.

A study carried out at Bayler University Medical Centre in Boston revealed that calcium in supplement form was absorbed as effectively as in milk products.

When considering any supplements the first rule is correcting the diet. Calcium is present in significant amounts in a very limited number of foods. Dairy products are probably the highest source of calcium but because of cholesterol problems, lactose intolerance and intact protein allergy, the recommendation that everybody should consume large quantities of dairy products could have other and more devastating effects on the community.

A well-balanced diet is the cornerstone of all good health and a variety of foods including fish, lean meats, raw vegetables and fruits, unprocessed brans and cereals should be included in everybody's daily dietary requirements. Foods such as chocolate, which contains oxalic acid, should be avoided when taking calcium as it may form other insoluble compounds that cannot be absorbed. Also large amounts of phytic acid present in cereals and grains may also inhibit absorption of calcium by the body.

Certain other factors influence the correct assimilation of calcium. It is very important to include weight-bearing exercise such as walking in your daily routine and to try to avoid excessive stress.

One serious consequence of long-term calcium deficiency for women is osteoporosis. It is an increased porosity of the bone in which the bone softens; a reduction in bone mass. Its cause appears to lie in the gradual bone loss that occurs in everyone with advancing age, but which is especially marked in women after menopause. This greatly increases the risk of fractures and it is therefore important to prevent bone weakening and halt its progress before fracture occurs.

Different studies have indicated that a sufficiently high calcium intake can reverse a negative calcium balance and thereby suppress bone loss.

A recent double-blind study undertaken in Denmark demonstrated that calcium supplements resulted in a significantly slower rate of bone softening in the total body-bone mineral content.

If you are going to take a calcium supplement to raise the dietary levels of calcium then one containing calcium and phosphorus, calcium phosphate, is necessary.

Calcium is actively transported through the absorbent cells of the small intestine with phosphate which is now known as the main synergist for absorption. In fact, phosphate appears to be a natural regulator of calcium absorption, promoting absorption at low calcium concentrations, but forming poorly absorbable polyphosphate complexes if calcium intake is excessive.

Absorption efficiency is generally 30 to 50%, but may be as high as 80%, depending on the types of food present, the need of the body for the mineral, and the presence of vitamin D. Vitamin D works with the parathyroid hormone to regulate the amount of calcium in the blood. It is extremely important in both the absorption and the utilisation of calcium.

The Division of Nutrition, Bureau of Foods, Drug & Administration, Department of Health, Education and Welfare, Washington DC, USA states:

"Animals and man have the ability to maintain calcium balance over a wide range of calcium intakes, provided the calcium/phosphate ratios are balanced."

Bio-calcium (available in health food stores) contains a natural form of calcium phosphate which is the most desirable form for both absorption and utilisation in the body.

Calcium absorption is highest when supplements are taken with a meal. Studies have shown that people with inadequate stomach acid have the same absorption of calcium as people with normal stomach acid production.

SUPPLEMENTS

calcium phosphate   2400 mg daily contains 720 mg
                               calcium

CANCER

Cancer can take many forms. Many studies report cancer could be an immune suppression or free radical disease, however, most cancers have one thing in common. Cancer cells form tumours which can destroy or compress other normal tissues. These malignant tumours are characterised by unrestrained cell growth and can spread to other parts of the body. Up to 25% of Australians may develop some type of cancer, however, it is important to remember that cancer is a word not a death sentence. Early detection and prompt treatment combined with natural therapies can make the difference between health and disease.

The possible signs and symptoms of cancer could be any one of the following:

1 Blood in your stool.

2 A mole which changes colour and size.

3 Coughing up blood.

4 A sudden change in bowel habits.

5 A persistent sore throat or change in timbre your voice.

6 An unusual lump in the female breast.

7 Persistent headaches and/or changes in vision.

If you have noticed any of the above do not panic. It may not be cancer. See your doctor immediately for further examination.

If cancer is the problem, putting it off will only make things worse.

To avoid cancer use commonsense. If you are smoking then the risk of lung and throat cancer is increased. This bad habit should be given up as soon as possible.

Your diet is vital. Do not eat food containing artificial colourings, flavours, preservatives, pesticides (cancer forming) or carcinogenic chemicals such as saccharine.

The diet must be high in fibre, whole grains and root vegetables. Fruits are very important. A combination of these foods should make up 75% of your total energy intake from foods.

Restrict your intake of animal fats in your diet. Your total fat intake should be 15% of your diet. Remember, fats have twice the amount of energy as protein and/or carbohydrate. The remaining 10% of your diet is protein and should be derived from lentils, nuts, seeds, fish, dairy products and lean meats. Research has shown that a balanced high fibre/low fat diet can prevent most colon cancers.

Include in your diet cruciferous vegetables such as cabbage, broccoli, brussel sprouts and cauliflower. A report in the America Journal of the National Cancer Institute (1 June 1990) stated that Indole-3 Carbinol, a chemical found in these vegetables reduces the risk of breast cancer by speeding up the metabolism of the female hormone oestrogen. Several other studies have shown that people with diets rich in these vegetables have lower rates of cancer than the general public.

Medical research has also found that the natural antioxidant nutrient beta-carotene, found in yellow and green vegetables may also help prevent cancer and reverse changes in cells that precede the development of cancer.

Dr Peter Greenwald, Director of the National Cancer Institute, Division of Cancer Prevention and Control, stated that people should be urged to eat foods rich in nutrients believed to have cancer preventing properties. These are vitamins A,C,E, B12, folic acid, beta-carotene, selenium and fibre. Evidence has shown that taking antioxidant supplements may help prevent such cancers as lung, breast, cervical, bladder, colon, oesophageal, stomach and skin.

Antioxidants are needed in our diets to help control free radicals, and these free radicals if uncontrolled, may be the cause of many cancers. To provide maximum protection against the free-radical disease in cancer a continuous supply of the antioxidant nutrients must come from our diet. Some antioxidant nutrients such as selenium are lacking in Australian soils and a lack of this and other antioxidants may decrease our bodies' natural protection process against cancer.

Fish oil and cancer

Further research has shown cancer may be prevented by supplementing the diet with fish oil. Dr Rashida Karmali, Associate Professor of Nutrition at Rutgers University, New York, has found that fish oil supplements suppress signs of developing cancer in women in high risk groups. Dr George Blackburn, Associate Professor of Surgery at Harvard Medical School, says that based on present knowledge, he would be dumbfounded if fish oil did not help thwart the spread of malignant cells in women who undergo breast cancer surgery. He believes the fish oil may strengthen their immunity, killing wandering cancer cells before they start new tumours.

Studies have shown that people who are dying from cancer have a low level of vitamin C in their diets and those ingesting large amounts of vitamin C reduced the possibility of developing cancer by 50%. Professor Linus Pauling found that in controlled studies 10000 mg of vitamin C taken orally each day by terminally ill patients increased their lives by up to one year more than expected.

As 60% of women's cancer and 40% of men's cancers are related to dietary factors, prevention and treatment of some cancers with diet and dietary supplements is very important and may indeed save lives.

SUPPLEMENTS

evening primrose oil   (may reverse carcinogenesis)
fish oil
antioxidant formula (vitamins A,C,E, zinc)
selenium
garlic   (supplement may inhibit tumour
beta-carotene   growth)
calcium phosphate
Lactobacillus acidophilus
Echinacea

10 Step anti-cancer plan

1 A diet balanced in low fat and high fibre.

2 Don't smoke.

3 Eat only organically-grown vegetables.

4 Maintain correct weight for height.

5 Reduce alcohol intake or stop altogether.

6 Don't sunbake and burn.

7 Supplement your diet with essential fatty acids and antioxidants

8 Avoid carcinogenic chemicals such as benzine, nicotine.

9 Reduce your stress levels.

10 Have a positive outlook on yourself and life.

CAFFEINE

Coffee and tea relate to many health problems, headache and heart disease being two. I would now like to examine these two beverages that most of us consume each day, and their side-effects.

Coffee stimulates gastric acid secretion which may lead to stomach ulcers. Many studies have been carried out over the years to determine if coffee increases the risk of heart attack. After reading many of these trials, I am personally convinced that it does. Many of the studies show that coffee increases serum cholesterol and is linked to hardening of the arteries (arteriosclerosis) and an increase in the risk factor for coronary heart disease. One trial in the *Lancet*, 1972, stated that heart attack was correlated with coffee but not tea consumption.

For information on headaches and coffee or tea, see Headaches. Caffeine seems to be the offender and coffee is more frequently associated with most problems.

I would recommend that if a choice between tea and coffee needs to be made, then tea is the better of two evils, but, why not try some of the herbal teas that are low in tannins and have no caffeine? This change will help reduce the risk of heart disease, headaches and ulcers and improve your quality of life.

CANDIDA (monilia)

Many women especially are suffering from candidiasis (infection with any species of *Candida*) and its associated side effects. One of the main causes of candidiasis in younger people is the use of antibiotics for skin disorders. These antibiotics unbalance the natural gut flora and diminish the normal levels of *Lactobacillus acidophilus* which is a friendly bacteria living in the intestine and needed for normal digestion. When it is at a low level then *Candida albicans*, a fungus also found in the small intestine, starts to multiply rapidly. Some of the indications of an infestation of *Candida albicans* are bloating, indigestion, flatulence, lethargy and thrush or redness, ulcers and irritation in either the mouth or genitals.

A diet that is low in sugar and refined carbohydrates is necessary. Too many dairy products and those containing yeast should be avoided. Quite often it is a problem diagnosing someone who has this complaint and all too often it is treated for its various effects rather than the cause. It is therefore very important to make sure you tell your doctor.

Write everything down that you feel is abnormal. This can be of great benefit in the ultimate diagnosis. New methods of detecting *Candida albicans* spores in the bloodstream, with dark field microscopic examination, are available. Stool counts can also be done, but one of the most reliable is the persistence of a number of symptoms and it has been shown that the analytical laboratory technique of examination will not always pick up this condition.

The dietary method of attack is to kill off any excessive *Candida albicans*. A high potency garlic supplement will do this. You need to recolonise the *Lactobacillus acidophilus* supplement. The powdered *Lactobacillus acidophilus* are extremely good and palatable but do not take the garlic and the *Lactobacillus acidophilus* together. The garlic should be taken at least three hours before *Lactobacillus acidophilus*.

It must be remembered that the prevention of recolonisation is a long-term treatment and it is not going to happen in one or two days so the ongoing garlic and *Lactobacillus acidophilus* supplement need to be continued until the symptoms disappear.

The inflamed and irritated orifices can be soothed with a diluted form of tea-tree oil which is a powerful anti-fungal and can kill off the *candida* infestation which is causing this problem.

Exercise and a positive outlook are also important as this stimulates the immune system and the metabolism, and it is a combination of all these things that lead to a positive result in the end.

The absorption of nutrients is affected by this breakdown in the normal gut intestinal flora. It is important to supplement your balanced diet with at least a multivitamin mineral preparation and it is a good idea to increase the vitamin C level to at least 2000 mg a day. The use of essential fatty acids is also important in the treatment, especially the monosaturated type such as olive oil and soybean oil. One teaspoon daily is recommended.

Vitamin C and zinc are essential in building the immune system and strengthening and revitalising the whole body. Following long-term *candida* infestation the immune system is weakened and unable to cope adequately with other infections at the same time as the *candida* infestation, so again the need for supplements is brought about. The herb, *Echinacea,* is also important here to help activate the immune system.

One of the most important things to remember is that a *candida* infection can be cured and that if you follow the diet, that is, a high roughage, complex carbohydrate diet, low in dairy products, low in yeast, with virtually no refined carbohydrates, then you will make it difficult for the *candida albicans* to flourish. Follow that with garlic to help knock down the infestation and recolonise with the *Lactobacillus acidophilus*.

SUPPLEMENTS

morning and night take

evening primrose oil	1 capsule 3 times daily
Bio ACE	1 morning and night
Echinacea	300 mg dried herb twice daily
garlic	2000 mg fresh herb twice daily

Lactobacillus acidophilus 4 hours after taking morning supplements.

Note: Garlic should not be given to infants.

CHILBLAINS

Chilblains are a common complaint that results from poor health and/or poor circulation in a damp, cold environment. Chilblains affect the extremities — the toes, fingers and ears. The symptoms range from itching to a burning sensation that soon becomes red, painful and swollen when in contact with heat. The person must be kept warm, the affected area must not be rubbed. Cocoa and soup will help restore circulation and no alcohol is to be consumed as it will aggravate the problem. Cigarette smoking also reduces the blood supply to the extremities.

Localised Treatment

One part of cayenne (chilli pepper),
one part of slippery elm powder, two parts vegetable oil.
Mix all these together and apply to affected area morning and night.

SUPPLEMENTS

see Cold Hands and Feet, Cold extremities, Smoking for cirulation.

CHILDREN AND MULTIVITAMINS (also see Hyperactivity)

Do children need vitamin supplementation? Can they function well on the diets they are currently receiving?

Do your children eat a lot of junk food? Children being children are known to spend their pocket money on junk foods at the local shop or leave their lunch in their school bag. Local take-away foods and junk foods are used more and more and the nutritious home cooked meal is left uneaten, the stomach already full with the chips or ice-creams that may have been eaten that afternoon after school. Eating from the five food groups each day is essential and a well balanced diet with wholegrains, fresh fruit and vegetables, dairy products, meats and/or protein substitutes such as nuts and lentils is important. We should ensure that our children are not eating an abundance of refined carbohydrates, sugar, fried foods, and food with artificial colourings and preservatives.

Exercise and a good night's sleep is a must if we want our children to grow up strong, healthy and happy. If you find that your children don't lead this lifestyle then a good multivitamin/mineral formula should be considered.

Modern medical evidence has now confirmed the benefits of multivitamin/mineral preparations for school children. A scientific study in Wales, in the British Isles, showed that the intelligence of children was improved by supplementing multivitamin/mineral formulations. This was reported in the British journal, *The Lancet*, in January 1988. A group of children was given a multivitamin and mineral supplement for a period of eight months and were compared with a similar group who were given a placebo. It was found that in the group taking the vitamin/mineral supplement there was a marked improvement in intelligence.

As well as a vitamin/mineral supplement, a chewable vitamin C tablet which is especially formulated for children's needs is a good idea. These supplements are recommended for children to help balance out any deficiencies and to give them the chance to reach their full potential for the times their diet may be inadequate.

SUPPLEMENTS

children's multivitamin formula as directed.

CHOLESTEROL

Cholesterol is a complex fatty substance made by the liver in all animals. It is very important and necessary for the formation of cell membranes and to help in the synthesis of bile acids, some hormones, and vitamin D. Only one-quarter of the body's cholesterol is obtained from the diet, the rest is manufactured by the body and because of this we must stay fit and pay particular attention to our weight. Modern studies have shown that overweight people produce 20% more cholesterol than people of normal weight for age.

There are five types of cholesterol, but it is the high density and low density cholesterol that we need to look at more closely.

The high density cholesterol or HDL, as it is commonly known, has the ability to clear built-up cholesterol from the arteries and help in its removal from the body. The low density of LDL is correlated with heart disease and could be responsible for fatty build up on the artery walls.

The good news is that if we have high blood cholesterol (over 5.5 millimoles per litre) for most of us, there are ways to bring it down.

1 We need to eat more cereal fibre such as oat bran, rolled oats, soybeans.

2 We need to cut down on our intake of all animal fats and increase our intake of polyunsaturated fats such as safflower, sunflower and soybean oils. No more than 30% of the total kilojoules in our diet should come from fats. Supplementing the diet with evening primrose oil (containing essential fatty acids) can also help lower cholesterol blood levels.

3 Exercise is also very important. It can raise the HDL cholesterol levels and burn up kilojoules. Around 30 minutes exercise three times a week is a good idea. Sports such as swimming, walking, skipping or bike-riding are excellent. Try to raise a light sweat — do not overdo it.

4 Evidence has now shown that taking garlic each day could help lower overall cholesterol blood levels and increase the levels of HDL over LDL cholesterol. Blackmores make a one a day low odour garlic called Garlix that could make taking garlic more sociable.

LOW CHOLESTEROL DIET

Any 1 or 2 choices of the following recipes for breakfast or lunch
  This plan is intended for persons wishing to attain or maintain a low blood cholesterol level. It should be noted that most Australians have a higher than average cholesterol level which may be dangerous as it can lead to increased heart disease and poor health.

MEAL INSTRUCTIONS:

1 The serving size depends on your level of activity.

2 If overweight, limit the serving size and increase your physical activity.

3 It is best not to use sugar but a little honey if needed.

4 No animal fats.

5 Choose no-or-low cholesterol foods.

6 No nuts, seeds, shellfish.

BREAKFAST:

Fruit: fresh whole fruit

Cereal: muesli, wheat cereals, bran, wheat germ plus skim milk or low fat yoghurt. Add two tablespoons of oat or rice bran.

OR

Eggs: A maximum of 2 eggs allowed weekly. You may eat extra egg whites only.

Bread: (whole grain stone ground) bread, crispbreads or rice crackers

Drinks: water, fruit juice, herbal tea, dandelion tea or coffee, skim milk.

DAILY MILK ALLOWANCE:

450ml low fat or 600ml skim/non-fat milk or soy milk, depending on your weight.

LUNCH:

Bread: whole grain, rice crackers.

Fillings: Salad, fish (tuna/salmon), low fat cheese such as ricotta or cottage cheese.

Mixed Beans: Any dried beans cooked in water such as soybeans, lima beans, broad beans.

Yoghurt: Low fat.

Vegetables: Any vegetable, steamed, not fried.

Fruit: Any fruit.

Drinks: Water, skim milk, fruit juice, mineral water and dandelion tea or coffee.

DINNER

Meat: Three lean red meat meals per week, cutting away all visible fat, avoid offal meats, casserole/stew is permitted but skim off fat.

OR

Chicken: Remove skin and grill or steam

OR

Fish:

Vegetarian Dish: Using soybeans or lentils, baked beans, dry peas, nuts, seeds or nutmeat.

EXTRAS: 1 to 2 slices wholegrain bread, salads, fresh fruit, low fat yoghurt or cheese

DRINKS: mineral water, water, dandelion tea or coffee.

SUPPLEMENTS

garlic (Garlix)	2000 mg enteric-coated dried herb take 1 tablet every morning with food.
evening primrose oil	take 1 capsule with meals 2 times daily
vitamin B3 (niacin)	slow release daily
dandelion tea	4 cups daily
oat or rice bran	1 tablespoon whole grain cereal every morning
psyllium husks	2 teaspoons in orange juice twice daily

Globe artichoke — Globe artichoke has been used for centuries and was known to medieval Arabic physicians. It stimulates liver function and cell regeneration and can help lower blood cholesterol. It is a delicacy and should be included in the diet.

CIGARETTE SMOKING

Smoking over the years has been an image maker, something to stop stress, or eating and putting on weight. When asked a difficult question, a cigarette can act like a child's thumb. It can be stuck in your mouth while you are thinking of an answer. The burning question is "*How can I give up Smoking?*"

One of the problems that you can suffer if you are a non-smoker is side-stream smoke. This side-stream smoke is the smoke that comes directly off the cigarette without passing through the filter. Most of us have, at one time or another, sat at a table with a smoker and noticed that the smoke coming from the cigarette seems to follow the same pattern as smoke from the fire when we are burning-off garden refuse. No matter where you stand, it always blows in your face. Side-stream smoke is dangerous. According to scientific investigation it has even more toxins than mainstream smoke or the smoke that the smoker inhales directly from the cigarette through the filter. As a smoker you are not only inhaling the mainstream smoke but at the same time you are inhaling the side-stream smoke, placing you at even higher risk.

Apart from the most feared danger of cancer, did you know that smoking can greatly affect the whole circulatory system?

The toxins, including nicotine, in tobacco have an effect on your arteries and veins causing constriction. This constriction is not unlike using a small garden hose garden to fill a swimming pool. There is just not enough water getting through to do the job. The same applies in your blood vessels if they are constricted. This can result in increased blood pressure, heart pain, increased ageing, or even gangrene of the legs. Smoking is known to cause heart disease, can increase your risk of cancer by 30%, will activate an early menopause which in turn accelerates osteoporosis, it affects hearing as supply of blood to the cochlea is reduced. Diabetics, sufferers of heartburn, and people with ulcers are all advised to give up smoking.

There are also a number of nutrients that are either destroyed or used up at a faster rate when smoking or when you are near a smoker. The most common of these is vitamin C.

There are a number of ways to give up smoking such as 'cold turkey' or gradual withdrawal. If you are one of the smokers who smoke 7300 cigarettes per year or 20 cigarettes per day, then smoking is one of your most frequently performed daily habits and giving up could be more difficult.

The best way to start is by juice fasting. Juice fasting helps the body cleanse itself by greatly increasing the cleansing and eliminating capacity of the lungs, liver, kidneys and skin. The digestive and elimination systems are not under such a strain and the accumulated toxins and metabolic waste is quickly eliminated from the body. This elimination juice-fast-diet also removes other toxins from the body taking away the desire to smoke cigarettes quickly.

In my clinic, a large number of patients who came to see me

for the first time were smokers trying to give up the habit. In conjunction with a juice fast, I have found that most people benefit from clinical hypnotherapy.

Dr Gary Duthie of Rowett Research Institute of Aberdeen, Scotland, reported on research that indicated smokers are under higher oxidant stress than non-smokers and that this stress can be partially compensated by vitamin E supplementation. A homeopathic smoke stop preparation can help take away the desire to smoke.

Calming the nerves can be done by taking a formula containing *passiflora*, scullcap, valerian and hops in combination with a B group vitamin formula. This combination will calm stressful nerves and take away the desire to smoke. You then need to repair the lungs with cod liver oil containing vitamins A and D plus essential fatty acids, combined with vitamins E and C.

SUPPLEMENTS

vitamin E	500 IU daily
vitamin C	2000 mg daily

COLD HANDS AND FEET (Raynaud's Syndrome)

Cold hands and feet can be very uncomfortable, especially in winter, but some people suffer this problem constantly. It is caused by an abnormal spasm of blood vessels.

This poor circulation in the extremities can be caused from smoking. It is a documented fact that smoking causes peripheral vaso-constriction which lessens the blood flow to the extremities. If you are smoking then you should stop.

The vitamins contained in your food especially vitamin E can be very important. Vitamin E helps improve circulation. Start with 100 IU of vitamin E daily and slowly increase over six weeks to 500 IU daily. Herbs such as hawthorn berry can be very beneficial. Hawthorn berries have the ability to help dilation of the blood vessels, especially in the extremities, and this vasodilation warms the hands and feet.

Ginkgo and garlic are herbs that can also improve circulation. Chilli peppers can be included with your food and will warm you up. Chillies can be in a tablet or capsule.

SUPPLEMENTS

vitamin E	500 IU daily
Ginkgo Plus Formula contains:	1 tablet morning and night
Ginkgo	500 mg
hawthorn	100 mg
garlic	250 mg
cayenne	30 mg dried herb daily
vitamin B3 (nicotinic acid)	up to 100 mg per day

COLD SORES — Herpes (genital and simplex)

Cold sores are a viral infection (*herpes simplex*) and are highly contagious. The name cold sores applies to their appearance when you are suffering with a cold. They can also accompany periods of stress. The reason they manifest at this time is because your immune system is underactive when you have a cold, an infection, or are under stress.

There are many things that can be done nutritionally to help prevent cold sores. Limit arginine which is an amino acid contained in protein foods. If the diet has a high arginine content and not enough L-lysine, which is another amino acid which is essential for growth and repair, then cold sores seem to proliferate. It is best to eliminate foods such as chocolate, which is very rich in arginine, and some of the red meats.

Taking a supplement containing zinc, vitamin C and L-lysine can be of enormous benefit. Research has shown that the combination of these nutrients can help prevent the recurrence of cold sores. The cold sore virus can lay dormant during periods of good health and low stress, so it is important to keep up the supplement and dietary program for at least three months.

Another herb that can help fight viral infections is *Echinacea*. It can help stimulate the immune system and is listed in the *British Herbal Pharmacopoeia* as an anti-viral herb.

The following supplements are also effective when used to treat *herpes genitalis* or genital herpes, cold sores on male and female genitals which are contagious and painful when present.

SUPPLEMENTS

Bio-C complex	1 tablet morning and night
zinc	25 mg per day
lysine	1000 mg per day
Echinacea	500 mg dried herb morning and night
garlic	2000 mg dried herb morning and night
tea-tree óil	apply 3 times daily

COLON CARE

The care of the lower bowel or colon is very important but unfortunately many of us neglect the inside. We need to drink plenty of water and eat foods high in roughage. Fresh fruits and vegetables and whole-grain foods are excellent and should be eaten every day in our diet.

We need to give our bodies a cleanout so that everything is functioning properly so we don't have any of the morbid wastes left behind that can quite often cause side effects such as headaches, or lethargy, or just not feeling up to par. Even cancer can result from not looking after our colon properly, and eating foods high in fibre.

To do this, we need to look after our colon with a Colon Care preparation, containing gentle laxative herbs and agents providing bulk. This will allow us to eliminate the toxins from our body and we should look at doing this periodically to make sure that we are keeping our colons healthy and flushed. It is very important to get rid of these toxins as they can cause many problems.

SUPPLEMENTS

High fibre diet	
Water	6–8 glasses a day
Colon Care contains	once every two weeks
cassia	
buckhorn bark	
psyllium seed	
aniseed	
fennel seed	
liquorice root	
uva-ursi	
Irish moss	
agar agar	

COMMON COLD AND FLU

There are many things we can do to help prevent the common cold and flu. Commonsense tells us to keep warm and out of sudden temperature changes from warm air conditioning to a cold day. Nutrition is also very important.

Recent studies (see Immune System) show that vitamin C can have a very helpful effect in helping prevent and/or reduce the symptoms of colds and flu.

We need to eat plenty of fresh fruit and vegetables and, as new scientific evidence suggests, a supplement to these 2000 mg of vitamin C each day is beneficial. A good form of vitamin C is one that contains ascorbic acid and the salts of vitamin C, sodium ascorbate, calcium ascorbate and bioflavonoids. These bioflavonoids occur naturally with vitamin C.

The herb, *Echinacea* is mentioned in the *British Herbal Pharmacopoeia* for its anti-viral properties. It stimulates the immune system and with garlic, destroys the invading bacteria and viruses.

The fatty acids in cod liver oil help reduce inflammation and make breathing easier. The vitamin A content helps strengthen the mucous membranes.

SUPPLEMENTS

Euphorbia	can be obtained in combination
Echinacea	
garlic	
liquorice root	dose: follow directions
Bio-C	1000 mg twice daily
cod liver oil	5 ml daily (adults)

CONSTIPATION (also see Bran)

Constipation can have many causes. Some people have a predisposition to irregular bowel movements from childhood. People who are anxious and fretful can become constipated. Lack of exercise is a common cause. People who fail to establish a regular time for bowel movements can become chronically constipated and should accustom themselves to a bulky breakfast and sitting on the toilet, to train the bowel.

Constipation can bring about many other problems apart from

the obvious inability to pass normal stools. Headaches, a feeling of nausea, or just being generally unwell can also be a result of constipation.

We must rid our body of toxins and the major process to remove these toxins is through our bowels, our urine and our skin. If any of these systems are affected or clogged, then we may reabsorb some of these toxins and this can cause us to feel unwell.

It is important that we maintain good eating habits. Roughage (fibre) is essential. You can get this fibre by eating whole cereal grains. Bran is very important. I have discussed bran and its importance in lowering cholesterol but it is also very beneficial in helping prevent constipation. Include whole cereals, fruits, vegetables, in your diet but most of all, to soften the stools and help flush the body of toxins, don't forget water. You should be drinking 6 to 8 glasses a day.

If you find that your problem is not solved even after doing all the right things with your diet, or if you have difficulty in eating correctly all the time, then natural laxative herbs can be very beneficial. Herbs such as cascara, senna and cape aloes in a combination can help solve the problem of constipation. These herbs will stimulate natural peristalsis (bowel movement). As with all laxatives, you should not use them all the time. Twice per week will normally help the problem.

SUPPLEMENTS

water	6 to 8 glasses per day
psyllium husks	2 teaspoons in orange juice each morning
peritone	1 or 2 tablets every second night if required
magnesium complex	1 tablet twice daily

CRACKING SKIN

Quite often skin cracks around the heels, the hands or even the corners of the mouth.

The cracking around the mouth, which is the epithelium tissue of the mucous membranes, is often caused by a deficiency in vitamin A. Cod liver oil is a good source of natural vitamin A. It also contains essential fatty acids which make a difference in helping to heal the cracking tissues. Vitamin B can also help and it is a good idea to take a vitamin B complex daily.

Cracking in the heels and the hands is often associated with occupation, for example, washing or working with feet in water. Detergents dry the skin out resulting in cracking. A *calendula* cream on the hands and the feet can help. *Calendula*, used for hundreds of years, is a soothing healing herb which also has antiseptic properties.

Other important essential fatty acids are found in evening primrose oil. Evening primrose oil has been well researched and has shown to be of benefit in the treatment of many skin disorders. Start with 6 capsules per day for 3 weeks then reduce to 2 capsules per day.

The mineral silica, although the most abundant of all minerals, may be lacking in the diet. Signs of silica deficiencies are cracking heels and weak, soft nails.

SUPPLEMENTS

fish oil 1000 mg	1 capsule 3 times daily
evening primrose oil	1 capsule 3 times daily
silica compound 25 mg Silica (celloid cell salt)	1 tablet morning and night
multivitamins and minerals	1 tablet daily
calcium fluoride 6x	1 tablet daily

CRAMPS (also see Menstruation)

Cramps are often associated with activities such as swimming. Cold water, poor circulation and cold weather conditions can also be the cause. However, there are many other causes of cramps, some of them related directly to our diet.

In the past we thought that salt was the answer. Troops during the Second World War were given salt tablets to help prevent cramps and it is quite possible that their poor diets were lacking in sodium chloride.

There is plenty of salt in all of our foods. A slice of bread, a daub of butter and any processed food will usually give us our daily requirement of sodium which is 200mg but quite often magnesium and calcium are lacking. A recent dietary survey of adults carried out by the Commonwealth Government showed us that these nutrients are lacking in most of Australian's diets.

Vitamin E can also help as it thins the blood and, along with helping improve circulation, increases the supply of oxygen to the muscles. A lack of magnesium will quite often bring about night cramps so taking a magnesium complex tablet could solve the problem and prevent those terrible knot-like cramps that can occur in your legs during the night.

SUPPLEMENTS

magnesium phosphate	200 mg twice daily
calcium phosphate	200 mg twice daily
vitamin E	250 IU daily
Ginkgo	400 mg twice daily

CROHN'S DISEASE

Crohn's disease, of unknown origin, is an inflammation of the bowel possibly from an immune defect. Studies now indicate that it is blocking of the small blood vessels feeding the intestine. Death of small sections of the bowel could be responsible for the ulceration and fissuring of the gastric mucosa.

In chronic cases the patients complain of pain mostly in the right-hand side of the gut, and of diarrhoea. During the acute stage weight loss, noticeable lack of energy, and sometimes fever and anaemia may be evident. Patients usually feel despondent and have a poor outlook on life.

The diarrhoea may be accompanied by pus, mucus and/or blood if the colon is affected. Seldom is there frank blood.

These are indicators that Crohn's disease and ankylosing spondylitis and ulcerative colitis may be linked in families sharing a common but incomplete genetic basis.

As the main medical treatment is corticosteroids there is the danger of acute adrenal insufficiency in patients treated with this drug. It may be brought about by the abrupt withdrawal of the corticosteroid or the patients' adrenals being unable to cope with increased infection or stress.

Prednisone and sulfasalazine are therapeutic. However, herbs and nutrients are used that have an anti-flammatory and vascular supportive action. Slippery elm, liquorice , omega 6 and omega 3 fatty acids (from fish oils), and evening primrose oil, with vitamin E can be used with medicine prescribed by the doctor. The combination is most beneficial. Refined sugar must not be taken as it contributes to increased inflammatory action for Crohn's disease sufferers. Hypoallergenic, low residue elemental diet is recommended. This reduces the load on the colon and vascular system in the gastrointestinal tract.

The omega 3 fatty acids in fish oil have anti-inflammatory effects. This is so for vitamin E which also reduces the viscosity of the blood. This vitamin improves blood flow and oxygen supply to the area, helping to prevent infarction of the colon. The vitamin E inhibits lukotriene formulation and reduces free radical damage because of its antioxidant properties.

Slippery elm, indicated for conditions of inflammation and ulceration as well as colitis, contains mucilage which is soothing to the gastrointestinal tract. Slippery elm is valuable when it is used with fish oil and evening primrose oil for the acute stage of Crohn's disease.

SUPPLEMENTS

vitamin E	1 capsule 3 times a day
slippery elm	600 mg 3 times a day
marshmallow root	500 mg 3 times a day
Lactobacillus acidophilus	2.5 billion bacilli once a day
multivitamin mineral	1 tablet a day

CYSTITIS

Cystitis is the inflammation of the bladder. The symptoms are usually a burning feeling during urination and a need to urinate frequently. The inflammation may be caused by a secondary infection in the urethra, the kidney, or by retained urine in the bladder caused by an enlarged prostate gland.

Cystitis is most common among women under 50 years of age, particularly during pregnancy. Sexual intercourse can lead to inflammation that can spread to the bladder by way of the urethra. This is often called 'honeymoon cystitis'. Poor hygiene and tampons can also cause inflammation.

If you are a frequent sufferer of cystitis there are a number of things that can be done to help prevent further attacks and relieve the symptoms.

1. Wear cotton underwear, never synthetic.

2. Drink 6 to 8 glasses of water daily. Water helps flush the kidneys, bladder, and urethra.

3. Eat alkali-forming foods (see list in acid/alkali food chart). All vegetables and fruits are alkaline after digestion and should be eaten every day. Your diet should be 80% alkali-forming foods and 20% acid-forming foods. Eating foods in these proportions will help maintain good health and prevent infection.

There are a number of herbs that can relieve the symptoms and clear up the infection quickly. They are corn silk, boldo marshmallow, couch grass and bearberry.

SUPPLEMENTS

buchu	440 mg 3 times daily
bearberry	
(*Arctostaphylos uva-ursi*)	230 mg 3 times daily
cornsilk	800 mg 3 times daily.
couch grass	800 mg 3 times daily
sodium sulphate	33 mg 3 times daily
sodium phosphate	195 mg 3 times daily
vitamin C	200 mg daily
vitamin E	500 IU daily

DANDRUFF AND ITCHY SCALP

If you are suffering from dandruff and itchy scalp then the first thing to do is to take regular care of your scalp by correctly washing it. You should look at washing your hair in a shampoo that suits your particular hair type. For instance, if you have oily hair, then you should use a shampoo containing wild nettle. Wild nettle is excellent for the removal of grease and oil without stripping the hair of its essential oils.

If you have medium hair and your scalp is itchy, then marshmallow is very soothing to inflamed membranes. If your hair and scalp are very dry then a mixture of almond and milk protein is excellent. This can strengthen the hair shaft and also solve a lot of the problems associated with dry scalp.

Rubbing Apricot E oil, which is a mixture of apricot kernel oil and vitamin E into the scalp can also be valuable as it helps bring the blood supply to the scalp and quite often cures dry scalp problems.

Essential fatty acids such as cod liver oil and evening primrose oil are good in the diet. Zinc helps maintain proper sebaceous gland function and therefore helps normalise the oil on the scalp and hair.

SUPPLEMENTS

cod liver oil   5 ml daily
evening primrose oil   500 mg 1 capsule 3 times daily
zinc   25 mg daily
multi vitamin/mineral   1 tablet daily

DIABETES MELLITIS (late onset)

Diabetes mellitis is a serious metabolic disease in humans resulting in an inability to metabolise carbohydrate, protein and fat. Your medical practitioner can perform blood and urine tests to examine the glucose (blood sugar) levels. If these levels are too high then special diets and/or medication may be required. If left untreated diabetes can lead to an increased risk in eyesight problems and cardiovascular disease.

There are five subclauses of diabetes mellitis and your medical practitioner is the only person who can determine your particular problem. If you have noticed a change in your vision, increased thirst or unexplained headaches it is important to see your practitioner and have a blood and urine test to rule out or confirm your suspicions.

Natural therapy has a lot to offer to sufferers of diabetes mellitis. Recent research has found that minerals, vitamins, and herbs combined with a high fibre, high complex carbohydrate diet can benefit. Chromium is a necessary part of glucose tolerance factor (GTF) and has been shown to increase glucose tolerance in animals, improving the effect of insulin. A good source of chromium is brewers yeast. Studies have also shown that glucose tolerance is improved when the diet is supplemented with chromium (see appendix).

The diet should be high in fibre and include cereal grains, legumes and root vegetables. The kilojoule intake of your diet should be 75 % from complex carbohydrates, 15 % from protein, and 10 % from fat. Refined sugar must be excluded.

Vitamin C can be of benefit as can the mineral zinc, as diabetics tend to excrete zinc in the urine. Essential fatty acids also help.

SUPPLEMENTS

GTF chromium yeast   as directed on the bottle
vitamin C   2000 mg or more daily
zinc   25 mg daily
multi vitamin   (sustained release) one daily
evening primrose oil   one three times daily.

DIARRHOEA

Diarrhoea can be caused by antibiotics, food poisoning, anxiety. Such attacks are usually short. Prolonged attacks indicate something more serious, such as a food allergy or a major disease of the colon.

Loss of fluid is a side effect and can be critical especially if your children are affected. Babies and very young children can be really at risk if they are suffering acute diarrhoea. If this is the case, then you must see your medical practitioner as dehydration can result.

If it is just loose stools or diarrhoea accompanying a cold, flu, or gastro-intestinal infection, then quite often there is something you can do about it.

When experiencing an attack of diarrhoea avoid eating dairy products. Diary products contain lactose and lactose can cause diarrhoea in lactose-intolerant people. Avoid oranges. These are known to exacerbate diarrhoea.

Eat foods that are dry. Dry biscuits or rice crackers help relieve symptoms. It is also important to keep up the fluids. Fluids sweetened with natural glucose are best. A herb to relieve diarrhoea is agrimony. Agrimony Complex is ideal to take and it is also safe for children.

For people who are anxious and suffer regular attacks of diarrhoea slippery elm can be taken in exactly the same way as it is for people who suffer constipation. It has been found to regulate people who have six or more bowel movements a day down to one or two.

SUPPLEMENTS

Herbal Complex containing:—
agrimony

kola extract
rhubarb root
slippery elm   follow directions on bottle
bayberry
mineral water with added glucose
rice biscuits
water 6–8 glasses per day

DIVERTICULITIS (irritable bowel syndrome)

Diverticulitis is inflammation of the diverticula. Irritable bowel syndrome is inflammation of the intestinal tract, especially the colon. These become inflamed and can be very painful, causing diarrhoea and cramping pains. If you have this problem you need to look at your diet and make sure that it is high in fibre. Don't skip meals especially breakfast. What you should be looking at is a daily intake of whole-grain cereals, fruits and vegetables. You must make sure you are drinking enough water as water softens the stools and can help relieve the pain.

An excellent fibre to use is psyllium husks. Psyllium seek husks can be mixed into a glass of orange juice and taken with breakfast. This ensures that you are obtaining a very soft fibre which is easily passed through the system.

There are also some herbs which can help, one of them being slipperly elm. slippery elm contains a mucilage which coats the gastro-intestinal track also helping to soothe the inflammation, relieving the problem.

SUPPLEMENTS

psyllium husks   2 teaspoons in orange juice once daily
slippery elm   600 mg of the powdered herb, just after
                            meals three times daily

Lactobacillus
acidophilus   2.5 billion bacteria daily
peppermint oil   0.2 ml daily

DIET

High fibre diet, mainly vegetable. Low animal fat and red meat. Eat five small meals, drink 6 to 8 glasses of water per day.

DRY SKIN

Continual skin care throughout life can improve the condition and texture of skin. Nutrition is of utmost importance for good healthy skin. Vitamin supplementation, especially vitamin E, is also important to help keep a healthy well-balanced skin.

If dry skin seems to be the problem then a proper skin care program should be implemented. It is essential for the skin to be cleaned by a product with gentle, soluble emollients and hand lubricating oils to offset the dehydrating effect of soaps. Almond cleansing cream has been specifically designed for this purpose.

Following cleansing, toning is important. One of the oldest yet most effective toners is witch hazel. This toner is an astringent which has a toning and anti-inflammatory effect. It contains natural oils, skin conditioner and moisturisers, so that the harsh effect of the toning is softened. This is an essential property in conditioners. Blackmore's Witch Hazel Toner is formulated to suit all skin types. A moisturiser containing a sunscreen is important. Probably one of the most valuable emollients and moisturisers is apricot kernel oil combined with soothing anti-septic and anti-inflammatory herbs such as fennel and chamomile. These herbs and oils have been combined in a product called Apricot Moisturising Day Creme with a natural sunscreen — PABA. This is an ideal nourishing, moisturising creme for daytime use and is excellent when used as a base.

A night moisturising program should be initiated. A richer moisturiser can be used with such ingredients as avocado and vitamin E. Avocado oil is a rich source of vitamins A, D, and E. Avocado oil is a rich source of vitamins A, D, and E and has a softening effect on hardened elastic skin tissue. It protects against dryness and chaffing. Vitamin E assists in skin repair and contracts the level of scar tissue. When combined with chamomile, mistletoe and yarrow, as in Blackmores Avocado Night Creme with E, then this is an ideal combination to nourish and moisturise which can be applied to the skin at night.

Exfoliation

Even though the skin is dry, the natural shedding process (exfoliation) still occurs and once a week it is a good idea to remove dead skin by using an exfoliation cream such as Blackmores Cinnamon Scrub which will gently scrub away the dead skin and open the pores to allow the skin to breathe freely making the skin healthy. It combines oatmeal and cinnamon, which are excellent cleansers, and honey for its soothing and healing properties, combined again with soy lecithin and lanolin as moisturisers and emollients.

So far we have just looked at caring for the face and neck but that is not the only part of our body which can be dry. We should then look at the whole body. The soothing properties of marshmallow and evening primrose oil can improve the skin. Marshmallow for general cleansing is very soothing to the skin and is an anti-inflammatory for problem skin. Marshmallow Complexion Soap will cleanse the skin without causing harshness or damage. Following that, a lotion containing evening primrose, applied over the whole body will soften, protect and nourish the skin.

A good hand cream containing calendula gives that extra protection for hands especially when associated with housework or work where the hands are exposed to detergents and cleansing agents.

SUPPLEMENTS:

evening primrose oil	1 capsule twice daily
cod liver oil	5 ml daily
antioxidant Bio ACE	1 tablet morning and night
(contains vitamins A,C,E and Zinc)	
silica compound	1 tablet morning and night

Use apricot kernel oil and vitamin E, or evening primrose body lotion

EPILEPSY

Epilepsy is a convulsive seizure. It affects people of all cultures. The disorder can be caused by changes in electric brain potentials or be hereditary.

The three types of epilepsy are, grand mal, petit mal and temporal lobe seizures.

Grand mal is the most well known. The sufferer may notice a change that can signal the arrival of the seizure. This change can range from a strange smell, flashing lights, ringing in the ears to feeling sick. This is then followed by a loss of consciousness, the sufferer then falls to the ground, the muscles are rigid, followed by shaking and twitching. There is also loss of bladder control, foaming at the mouth and blueness around the lips. The sufferer then falls into a deep sleep. The attack usually only lasts a few minutes.

Petit mal is a form of epilepsy that mostly affects children. These seizures only last a few seconds, usually no more than half a minute.

The symptoms of a petit mal seizure is usually a blank stare that may or may not be accompanied by rapid blinking. These attacks can occur many times daily, the sufferer does not lose consciousness and resumes normal activity straight after the attack.

Petit mal rarely affects adults.

Modern medicine has developed medicines such as Dilantin, Mysoline and Zarotin. These medications have made normal life possible for many sufferers of epilepsy. Naturopathic medicine has also a lot to offer the epileptic. Recent research published in the *Medical Journal of Australia* states that vitamin E supplement can reduce the number of seizures. Westmead Hospital researchers found that 8 out of 12 epileptic adults and 2 out of 6 children responded well to vitamin E supplement.

The herb scullcap, which is an anti-convulsive herb is useful when used in combination with *lupulus*. Scullcap also combines well with hops and passion flower for this condition.

There is considerable evidence that a low allergy diet is beneficial. Observation studies have shown that magnesium, manganese and zinc concentrations in the blood were lower in epileptic children. These same studies suggested that supplements may be beneficial. Adding the amino acids taurine and dimethyl glycine to the diet have also shown good results. Note: Epilepsy is a condition that is managed well by your medical practitioner. It is important not to discontinue any medication.

SUPPLEMENTS

vitamin E	500 IU 1 capsule twice daily
scullcap	500 to 1000 mg 3 times daily
magnesium phosphate	100 mg 3 times daily
zinc	1 tablet daily
taurine	500 mg 3 times daily
glycine	100 mg daily

vitamin B6(4)   100 mg daily
potasium chloride
   (celloid)   65 mg 3 times daily

EYES AND NIGHT VISION (See Night Vision and Eyesight)

FOOD ALLERGIES (See Allergies)

FASTING

Always contact your practitioner before going on any fast, or radical change to your diet.

The following juice fast has been designed to clean the body of toxic waste which has been accumulating in the tissues for many years. It is very important to include an enema in conjunction with your juice fast because without it the toxic waste and morbid matter which has been accumulating in your body cannot be flushed out. It remains in your colon where re-absorption could cause poisoning to your whole system.

The enema should be used a minimum of once per day. Preferably twice, once in the morning and last thing at night.

Prepare yourself for the fast by eating raw vegetables and fruit for 2 days before.

On the night before the fast take ONE teaspoon of colon care with a glass of water before bed. Use only purified water, not tap water.

This is a four day fast and the following fast advice should be carried out each day:

1 Upon rising drink a glass of fresh water then using 600 ml of warm water, give yourself an enema. Follow this by having a massage, if possible. If not, then a spa or high pressure hot and cool shower.

2 9.30 am   Cup of herbal tea, no milk or sugar

3 11.00 am   Glass of fresh water

4 11.30 am   Large glass of fruit juice diluted 50/50 with fresh water, not tap water. Take a short walk, have another massage or lightly exercise

5	1.30 pm	Large glass of vegetable juice
6	2.00 pm	Glass of herbal tea or fresh water
7	2.00 pm	Have a rest, *no exercise*. Take a relaxation class if you can at 4.00 pm or meditate
8	6.00 pm	Light walk and a bath with Epsom salts
9	8.30 pm	Glass of fruit juice Your intake of fluid should be a minimum of 8 glasses per day. This can include mineral water, herbal teas, and fruit juice.

When ending the fast it is important to introduce the normal diet slowly over 3 to 4 days beginning with a day of fruit and vegetables.

FLUID RETENTION

Many people, especially women, suffer with the problem of fluid retention. For women, just before menstruation, fluid is retained, breasts can be painful, and ankles and fingers can become swollen.

If you suffer with this problem of fluid retention then look at diet. Consuming too much sodium chloride, or salt, can lead to fluid retention.

Drink more water. Many people think that if you drink water you will retain more and more fluid. This is not the case. Drink 6 to 8 glasses a day. Many foods included in our diets are natural diuretics. Celery is one, cucumber is another, even apples are slightly diuretic, so include plenty of fresh fruits and vegetables in your diet.

Take herbs which have diuretic properties. They include celery seed, juniper berries, dandelion leaf and parsley piert. Juniper can irritate the kidneys and should not be taken if suffering from any kidney infection. Juniper is also contra-indicated in pregnancy. Dandelion is not irritating to the kidneys.

The vitamin B6 and the mineral sodium phosphate are nutrients that have diuretic properties and can help remove excess fluid. Vitamin B6 is of particular value in the treatment of pre-menstrual fluid retention.

SUPPLEMENTS

celery and juniper formula	2 tablets 3 times daily or as directed
herbal diuretic formula (based on dandelion)	1 tablet 3 times daily 1500 mg
vitamin B6	25 mg daily
water	6 glasses daily
Low sodium diet	

GALLSTONES (cholelithiasis)

This is a complaint which mainly affects the middle-aged and overweight. Women have four times the incidence of gallstones than men. Although the cause of this condition is not fully understood the disease is likely to be a metabolic disorder and probably related to diet.

Gallstones may be present without any symptoms. However, if a stone moves it may obstruct the common bile duct or neck of the gallbladder and this can result in agonising pain radiating from the upper right side of the abdomen through to the back and right shoulder.

Other symptoms which may indicate the presence of gallstones are a rapid pulse, pain or discomfort after eating fatty meals, mild jaundice and/or excessive flatulence. A complete blockage of the common bile duct is a medical emergency as it may develop gangrene.

It is important to restrict the intake of fat. Fat requires bile salts that are stored in the gallbladder for assimilation into the body and their ingestion can precipitate an attack.

Also cabbage, turnips, Brussel sprouts, cauliflower and broccoli are gas-forming and can increase the risk of cholelithiasis.

The naturopathic treatment for gallstones is prevention.

SEVEN STEPS IN THE PREVENTION AND CURE OF GALLSTONES

1 Eat a well-balanced diet that is low in animal fat (most gallstones are composed of cholesterol found in animal fat).

2 Include in the diet pears as they have a healing effect on the gallbladder.

3 Supplement the diet with lecithin. Lecithin increases the

phospholipid concentration in the gallbladder. Phospholipid concentration is known to be lower in patients with gallbladder disease.

4 Use a little olive oil each day on salads or to mash potatoes. Olive oil will stimulate the flow of bile helping flush out small stones as well as stimulating the production of the fat-splitting enzyme lipase. Maintain correct weight for height. Most gallstone sufferers are overweight.

5 Drink 4 cups of dandelion tea each day. Dandelion not only helps prevent gallstones but can dissolve them. Dandelion action is twofold. First, by direct effect on the liver, causing an increase in the flow of bile and, second, by direct action on the gallbladder causing contractions that force out stored bile and small (gravel) stones. This increase in bile flow also increases the amount of chendeoxycholic acid, an acid found in bile that over a period of time will dissolve gallstones.

6 Supplement with vitamins C & E. A number of experimental studies have also shown that if vitamin C and E are deficient in the diet there is a decreased level of bile acids, making the formation of gallstones more likely. Also cholesterol stones in vitamin-deficient animals dissolve when given vitamin E.

7 Eliminate symptom-provoking foods. Experimental studies have shown that eggs are the most common offender, however individuals differ. It is therefore important to establish which foods provoke symptoms.

I have used this formula with very good results. Ultrasound examination has shown that gallstones have been removed using the above program in many patients.

There are other methods such as gallstone flushing using vegetable oil, lemon juice and apple cider vinegar. This method is also successful, however if the gallstone is too large it may block the bile dudct and this could be dangerous. I would not recommend this method unless under the care of your practitioner

SUPPLEMENTS

SS 69, sodium sulphate
celloid cell salt   1 tablet 3 times daily
dandelion   1500 mg dried herb twice daily
olive oil   5 ml twice daily
lecithin (granules)   2 tablespoons daily

multi-B vitamin complex	1 daily
apple cider vinegar	1 teaspoon each morning with a little water and honey
vitamin E	500 IU daily
vitamin C	2000 mg daily

GARLIC

From ancient times, history around the world records the use of garlic for treating a whole range of health complaints. The Greeks and Romans wrote of its many beneficial effects, including being a wonderful aid to digestion and general health. Ancient Chinese, Indian and Egyptian records proclaim its benefits for respiratory disease, flatulence, dandruff, retarding ageing and treating high blood pressure. Roman gladiators took garlic to increase strength. In World War I the raw juice was expressed, diluted with water and put on swabs applied to wounds as an effective antiseptic.

Modern scientific research backs up garlic's long and glowing history. We now have ample evidence pointing to the benefits of taking garlic for lowering cholesterol and blood pressure, preventing coughs and colds, treating infections, sinus and bronchial problems and maintaining well-being.

What is it that makes garlic such a valuable herb? Its wide health-producing action seems to come from many ingredients, one of which is allicin. Allicin can inhibit the growth of bacteria and fungi which are harmful to the body. It also is an effective antiseptic and an excellent tonic supporting the immune system.

Of course, fresh is best and the raw garlic clove contains all the benefits (remember cooking reduces its effects), but eating it raw is often inconvenient, impractical and certainly unsociable! The next best thing is to use garlic in its freeze-dried form. This is the best way to guarantee that you will get all the benefits as the allicin may be damaged by heat, fermentation, processing, ageing or by addition of chemicals.

Garlic can also help balance the intestinal flora by inhibiting Candida which is a fungal-type infection sometimes characterised by uncomfortable symptoms such as bloating, wind, indigestion, thrush and sugar cravings. Here too, the versatile garlic may be the answer. However, to take full advantage of the antibacterial and antifungal effects of garlic in the intestine where it is needed to combat this problem, we need to be taking a garlic supplement protected in a special enteric coating so that the garlic is not absorbed or altered by the body before it reaches its target area (the intestine).

Garlic has a very beneficial effect upon many parts of the body. It is able to lessen the pain and discomfort of sinus problems, as well as helping to dry excessive mucus production. In the blood it has been seen to reduce the stickiness of platelets, hence reducing the risk of blood clots. It can also be used to help lower cholesterol levels and high blood pressure.

If you can't seem to shake that flu or just manage to get over one cold before another one descends, perhaps you need to help your Immune System along with a herb that not only has stood the test of time but is now proven, through scientific study, to be a true friend in sickness and in health.

GOUT OR CRYSTAL ARTHRITIS

Gout is a disease that can affect any person and can be a very painful affliction. Gout is the formation of uric acid crystals in the joints. These crystals cannot develop without an elevated level of uric acid in the blood, therefore, the prevention of this elevated level of uric acid is what needs to be treated.

In orthodox medicine prescription drugs are given to reduce inflammation and pain for acute attacks and/or the use of drugs such as allopurinol to reduce the amount of uric acid in the blood and urine.

The naturopathic treatment is based on the modification and reduction of the main factors that increase the uric acid levels in the blood.

THE DIET

A diet low in fats and moderate in the intake of protein is the first step in reducing uric acid levels in the blood.

Foods that contain a high level of purine should be avoided. These include all organ meats: ie liver, kidney, brains, heart, sweetbreads. Other foods that must be avoided are shellfish: prawns, lobster, oysters, salami, pate, sardines in oil, anchovies. Do not eat tomatoes or oranges. You can eat milk, eggs, cereal (except whole wheat), fruit, enriched bread, butter and most vegetables. Restrict to twice a week asparagus, beans, peas, alcohol, mushrooms, oatmeal, whole-wheat cereal.

To avoid rises in uric acid level do not take aspirin. Sudden changes in weight can cause a rise so weight reductions or increases should be gradual.

The consumption of red meat is to be restricted to three times weekly. Chicken and fish can be eaten freely but they must be grilled or steamed. Tomatoes, alcohol, take-away foods such as Chinese must be avoided.

It is also important to increase the amount of fluid intake to 6 to 8 glasses per day. Low purine diets are lower in Vitamin B, and a B Complex should be taken.

SUPPLEMENTS

B complex	1 tablet/capsule daily
vitamin C	5000 mg daily
pantothenic acid	50 mg daily
	alfalfa, juniper berries, parsley, celery seeds, potassium, silica
cod liver oil	5 ml daily

HAWTHORN (also see Blood Pressure)

Hawthorn (Crataegus monogyna) is a familiar tree in Europe, Asia and North Africa. It can grow to a height of about 9 metres with spreading thorny branches. The hawthorn flowers spring to mid-summer with white flowers, each producing a separate fruit which, when ripe, is a bright red colour.

The wood of the hawthorn is very hard and was used to make such articles as combs and small boxes. It was also used in Germany to divide the land into smaller parcels or plots. The word *haw* is an old name for hedge and also the word for the berry.

One can find Hawthorn growing along parts of the New England Highway in NSW and I have regularly harvested the ripened fruit, or haw, for use in my own clinics.

Fruit, either fresh or dried, is used as a cardiac tonic, diuretic, sedative and coronary vasolidator. Although widely used in eastern medicine as a sedative, diuretic, cardiac tonic and astringent, it has not been used in orthodox western medicine to any great degree. The native Americans used it to treat rheumatism.

The main constituents of hawthorn are Vitamin C, flavone

glycosides, catechins, saponins and other unidentified properties. It is the combined effect of the above constituents that gives hawthorn its medicinal uses. Scientific investigation has found that hawthorn can be useful in the treatment of many cardio vascular complaints.

Tests were carried out in Germany in the 1950's with reference to its use in conjunction with digitalis in the treatment of mitral stenosis. The results of these tests were generally beneficial. The patients with mitral stenosis were given hawthorn as a liquid extract. This form of medication proved to be successful and notable improvement was shown. It was also noted that those patients who were receiving digitalis drug therapy were able to discontinue the digitalis or considerably reduce the dose. Because of its ability to dilate the coronary heart vessels, hawthorn is an invaluable herb in the treatment of angina pectoris, high blood pressure, myocarditis, paroxysmal tachycardia and cardiac arrhythmias.

In my clincal practice I have use hawthorn in different and various combinations. In combination with garlic and *Cereus grandiflorus,* it has proved extremely beneficial in the treatment of high blood pressure. A patient who comes to mind first saw me with a systolic of 180, a diasystolic pressure of 100 and a blood cholesterol level of 6.5 mm/1. The patient was a male, 40 years of age, slightly overweight, who complained of thumping in the chest at night which was keeping him awake. In conjunction with his medical practitioner, I placed the patient on a low salt diet with a combination of hawthorn dried berries (500 mg), garlic (200 mg of the dried bulb) and *Cereus grandiflorus* (40 mg 3 times daily with meals), for a period of 3 months. With continual monitoring, it was noted that not only had the patient's blood pressure been reduced to 125/85, but the palpitations he was experiencing had completely disappeared. On examination of his cholesterol level, it was noted to have dropped from 6.5 mm/1 to 4.00 mm/1.

I have also used hawthorn in combination with a d-alpha tocopherol, for the relief of angina pectoris, on a number of patients. Because the ischaemic pain related to angina pectoris is a consequence of inadequate oxygenation of the myocardium, the ideal treatment of this condition would be to increase the blood flow in the coronary vessels and at the same time, decrease the myocardial requirement for oxygen.

As hawthorn is able to increase the flow of blood through the mycordium by dilating the coronary arteries (first observed by Ullsperger in 1951) and because hawthorn is a mild sedative, helping the patient to cope with the worry about their heart and the gripping pain that may come at any moment, it is an excellent herb to add to any cardiac formula.

The addition of d-alpha tocopherol (Vitamin E) to this formula is also valuable. It is a powerful fibrinolytic agent and antioxidant preventing the available oxygen in the blood from being converted into toxic peroxides. This action leaves the red blood cells with more oxygen and this of course, increases the availability of oxygen for the myocardium, resulting in a reduction of pain.

HAYFEVER

When spring approaches many people suffer from a number of allergy symptoms. One of the most common is spring hay fever, or allergic rhinitis. This is quite a devastating problem because if it becomes chronic, it can sometimes weaken the body's resistance and make it more susceptible to other diseases.

Airborne pollens including wheat and corn, fungi, spores and rusts can cause irritation of the mucous membranes in the nose and throat. This irritation can lead to a running nose and quite often sneezing attacks, along with a sore, itchy throat and itchy, swollen eyes. Spring hay fever differs from that of perennial allergic rhinitis which is not seasonal. It is brought by things like house dust, foods, feathers, industrial fumes, drugs and polluted air. Unfortunately most of us at one stage or another are subjected to these irritants and quite often experience the discomfort of sneezing attacks and congested and inflamed mucous membranes in the nose. What we have to do is find a way of preventing this annoying condition.

Remove things containing feathers such as eiderdowns from the house as these are known to cause problems. The house should be well ventilated and cleaned with a vacuum cleaner which has a micro-filter that prepares airborne particles of house dust returning to the air. Do not eat foods you may be allergic to. Dairy products can be a problem. Avoid growing plants that are proven allergens. Privet should not be grown and is restricted by law in certain states. If the problem still persists then look at what can be done to alleviate it.

It is interesting to note that medicine in the 1930s suggested cocaine be used to deaden the nostrils as a solution to this problem. Of course the symptoms and side effects of that certainly make this a remedy we would not even consider today but there are some herbs and vitamins that can have an effect in reducing the symptoms of allergic rhinitis.

The herb garlic can be of great value especially when combined with horseradish. Both of these herbs have a bacteriostatic or antibiotic action. Garlic has an expectorant and drying effect on the sinuses. Along with its bacteriostatic and antiseptic properties, it can be extremely helpful for sinusitis. The horseradish acts in promoting discharge and drainage of that area and is aso quite a powerful antiseptic. Combined with these, cod liver oil and extra vitamin A can be of benefit.

A combination of horseradish and garlic tablets, vitamin C complex, containing 1000 mg of a combination including calcium ascorbic acid, citrus bioflavonoids, rutin, hesperidin, rosehips and acerola, should be taken three times daily. To help build resistance, vitamin A (10,000 IU) in conjunction with the above, taken daily, can certainly have an effect in strengthening the mucous membranes, building resistance, drying out sinuses, and helping alleviate the problems of the spring hay fever or allergic rhinitis.

SUPPLEMENTS

Sinus and Catarrh formula	3 times daily
a herbal formula containing:	take 3 daily
horseradish, garlic, echinacea,	
liquorice root	
sambucus	100 mg 3 times daily
Bio-C	1000 mg daily
cod liver oil	5ml daily

HEADACHES

Migraine headaches are discussed under Migraines, but now let us look at so-called normal headaches. These headaches can develop after a hard day's work, or spending too much time in glary conditions. These are a different type of headache but certainly painful and debilitating.

There are a number of causes of headaches that are not migraines, for instance, if you drink alcohol, this depletes the body of vitamin B1 and dehydrates the brain which can lead to headaches. Many people, if they are drinking alcohol to excess, do suffer these headaches. So, consider a vitamin B supplement and keep up the fluids (non-alcoholic), if this is the case. However, it would be better to lower or stop your consumption of alcohol.

Food allergies can also cause headaches (see allergies). Removing the foods from the diet which are a problem may just solve all your headache problems.

Caffeine intake (found in coffee and tea) is related to headache. A study of 4558 Australians showed that caffeine intake significantly increased headaches. Even those ingesting 4 to 5 cups of coffee or tea daily (containing 250 mg caffeine) had a relatively higher risk of headaches. If coffee or tea is your problem, then consider reducing your daily intake but, remember, caffeine withdrawal has also been shown to cause headaches, leaving you with a 'catch 22' situation. The answer is slow reduction of caffeine intake. Reduce your coffee or tea consumption by one cup per day for the first week, then two cups for the second week and so on. This should then prevent caffeine-withdrawal headaches.

Headaches can also be caused by stress and strain. If a muscle is strained when lifting heavy objects then the neck muscles become knotted and painful. This pain travels up into other muscles in the head and becomes quite unbearable. You then have to resort to strong analgesics.

Consider relaxation, meditation, massage or using the herb valerian. This can help relax your tense muscles and prevent them from getting to the stage where you need to take strong analgesics to alleviate the pain.

If an analgesic is needed then don't forget the natural analgesic white willow bark as well. It is very effective (see analgesics).

Betony can also be used for specific forms of Headaches and neurasthenia such as those associated with stress and tension.

Also see Allergies.

SUPPLEMENTS

white willow bark (nature's aspirin)	5400 mg 3 times daily
vitamin B complex	1 tablet daily
and	
valerian	Can be obtained in
hops	combination
scullcap	
passiflora	Follow directions

HEART DISEASE

Did you know 26.3% of Australians died in 1988 of coronary heart disease and another 10.4% died from strokes? (National Heart Foundation 1988 'Heart Facts).

When you consider that heart disease is largely preventable, we really must be doing something wrong.

The heart is not the fragile organ most of us are led to believe. It is a very strong muscle about the size of a man's fist which sits in the middle of the chest. Without our heart the blood would not circulate around our bodies. This fantastic organ, beating at more than 100,000 beats per day, pumping about half a cup of blood per beat, pumps around 200,000,000 litres of blood in the average lifetime.

If you car worked as hard as your heart, then it probably would not last the distance, so those of us who just cannot afford to keep buying new cars do something about this problem. We keep up regular services, make sure the correct petrol and oil are used, warm our engines up slowly and do not over-rev them.

Do we give our hearts the same attention and loving care, taking into account the above figures? The average answer would be no, we do not.

A number of my patients come in to see me with this standard question: 'My father died from a heart attack when he was only 48 years of age and now my brother has developed angina. Does this mean that I am next and if so, if there anything I can do?

The answer is that family history only plays a small part in heart disease and a change in other risk factors can make all the difference. You are in a high risk group if you have high blood pressure, smoke more than 15 cigarettes a day, have high cholesterol, are overweight, live a stressful lifestyle or have diabetes. You must seek you practitioners advice and have a full medical check-up.

HOW TO PREVENT HEART DISEASE 8 STEP PLAN

1 Exercise for 28 minutes at least three times a week raising your heart rate to 80% of the maximum heart rate for age. (Maximum heart rate for age is 220– your age ie. If you are 40, 220–40 = 180, 80% of 180 is 144 beats per minute]).

2 Include fish oil in the diet. Fish oil contains omega 3 fatty acids that may be beneficial in protecting against the development of heart disease.

3 Eat a low cholesterol, well-balanced diet, high in fibre and low in animal fat. This can help prevent hardening of the arteries, one of the main causes of high blood pressure, strokes and heart disease.

4 Supplement the diet with vitamin E. Dr Wilfrid Shute and his brother Dr Evan Shute of Canada have used vitamin E for the treatment and prevention of heart disease and stated that 'the time has come when it should be pointed out that the average cardiologist can do nothing to help a damaged heart if he does not use Vitamin E except to treat symptoms and complications.'
Dr H. Esterbauer of the University of Graz, Austria, reported that vitamin E could help prevent atherosclerosis. Vitamin E also increases HDL cholesterol and reduces platelet adhesiveness.

5 Include garlic in the diet either by taking a garlic supplement or by eating it with your food. (A good garlic supplement is Garlix. It contains the freeze-dried herb with a natural enteric coating. This passes through the stomach into the intestine where it is absorbed without making the bad breath smell of garlic.) Garlic can help lower blood pressure and cholesterol. It may also help prevent hardening of the arteries.

6 Don't smoke: cigarette smoke causes vaso-constriction that can increase blood pressure, cause heart disease and cardiac arrythmias.

7 Learn to relax. Don't build up aggression. Take up a hobby and make time for yourself. Aggressive fast-living people have a higher incidence of heart disease.

8 Maintain the correct weight for height. Being overweight reduces your fitness and increases the load on your heart.

9 Eat high fibre, low animal fat foods (see cholesterol diet).

SUPPLEMENTS

multi-vitamin mineral	1 daily
vitamin E	500-1000 IU daily, start with 100 IU daily
Fish Oil 1000	1 capsule 3 times daily
evening primrose oil	1 capsule 3 times daily

garlix	1 tablet each morning
magnesium phosphate	100 mg twice daily
lecithin	1 to 2 tablespoons pure granules daily

HEALTHY NAILS

Quite often we overlook the importance of healthy nails and hair. These are signs, or can be signs, of ill health or dietary deficiencies.

What we should look for is unusual nail shape. If we have 'spoon' shaped nails this can indicate an iron deficiency. White spots on the finger-nails could indicate a zinc deficiency. These are very important minerals and quite often overlooked. Fatty acids which are found in evening primrose oil and fish oils are very important as well. These can help strengthen the nails.

Another mineral is silica. Silica is the most common mineral on our planet and yet you won't find it in most multi-vitamin preparations available. The addition of silica to the diet will strengthen your nails and hair.

SUPPLEMENTS

multi vitamin mineral formula containing iron, PABA, and zinc	1 daily
silica	50 mg daily
evening primrose oil	500 mg 1 capsule twice daily
fish oil	1000 mg 1 capsule twice daily

HEPATITIS (see Liver)

HERPES (see Cold Sores)

HOW TO LOSE WEIGHT

If we are overweight then as we get older, it can exacerbate many diseases such as osteoarthritis. Even cholesterol is increased in those who are overweight. It also can lead to blood pressure problems.

Eating correctly and having a well-balanced diet are very important. We should look at low fat foods and low calorie foods. Include celery, cucumber, and carrots as these are very low in calories, quite good snack food and also act as diuretics.

Evening primrose oil and alfalfa are excellent supplements. They help break up the fats and will help you lose weight.

To curb hunger pains try apple fibre with a large glass of water half an hour before your meal. Remember it is also very important to drink 6 to 8 glasses of water per day. If you do all of these things you will notice you will feel better and the weight will come off.

HYPERACTIVITY and CHILDREN

Some children appear to be overactive, running around the place much more than others of their age. Often parents ask, "Is hyperactivity a real thing?"

If your child is a lot more active than s/he should be and s/he suffers a lot of mood changes and is very hard to get along with there is a strong chance s/he is hyperactive.

This hyperactivity is diet-related. Certain foods need to be excluded from the diet. These include sugar and refined carbohydrates. Sugar is a known cause of hyperactivity.

However, often it is an allergy problem. We should look at food labels to see if they contain artificial colourings, flavourings and preservatives and remove them from the diet. This is really a case where fresh is best. You will still be able to give your child a treat by giving them something wholesome. They will get used to the change and they will be nowhere near as hyperactive as they were.

Salycilates (the main constituent of aspirin and found in many fruits) can be an allergen causing reactions. If your child is allergic and you suspect this is a cause then a cytotoxic blood test can confirm this. If the result is a problem then go on a low salycilate diet.

SUPPLEMENTS

children's multivitamin formula
Nervaid formula
scullcap, passiflora, hops, valerian (in combination)
dose as for age formula — a child under age of 12

$$\frac{\text{child's age in years}}{\text{age} + 12} = \% \text{ adult dose}$$

potassium phosphate   100 mg twice daily
magnesium phosphate   100 mg twice daily

HYPOGLYCAEMIA (Low Blood Sugar)

Many people in this modern world are suffering from functional hypoglycaemia. The symptoms of their complaint include headaches, loss of short term memory, dizziness and lassitude. The cause is usually the consumption of refined carbohydrates (sugar) in excess over a long period. This excess amount of sugar in the diet gives a short term lift (high energy) associated with the increase in blood sugar (glucose). However, their body reacts quickly to this increase and in the hypoglycaemic person, over-reacts. This overreaction reduces the blood sugar below what is needed for normal bodily function and can result in one or more of the above symptoms. These symptoms can be relieved by taking sugar, however, the process repeats itself and the symptoms soon return.

Changing the diet is the first step towards balancing blood sugar levels. Experimental studies have shown that a diet low in refined carbohydrates and fat and slightly higher in protein will, in time, return blood sugar levels to normal permanently.

Supplements may also be of benefit. Experimental double-blind crossover studies have shown that chromium supplement can alleviate the symptoms of hypoglycaemia within three months. Magnesium may also reduce glucose-induced insulin secretion. Supplementing could be of benefit and I have found in my clinic that the combination of diet and a supplement of chromium and magnesium has totally relieved all the symptoms of hypoglycaemia in patients.

A low refined carbohydrate diet, no added sugar in drinks or in foods (this will only make the problem worse), less fat and an increase in protein intake, is a recommended diet.

SUPPLEMENTS

magnesium compound	1 tablet 3 times daily
Bio Chromium from your practitioner or a chromium supplement containing	
GTF chromium yeast	1 tablet morning and night

IMMUNE SYSTEM AND VIRAL INFECTIONS

Viral infections and suppressed immune systems are of a greater problem today than they were in the 1960s and 1970s. Diseases such as Acquired Immune Deficiency Syndrome (AIDS), Chronic Fatigue Syndrome (CFS) and viral infections, are presenting practitioners and the public with symptoms not previously encountered.

Modern allopathic medicine has no answer to many of these problems and therefore many people are looking to natural therapies for answers.

One of the most common herbs used by the ancients and modern herbalists for the treatment of infection is *Allium sativum* (garlic). Garlic is a member of the lily family and it contains a volatile oil composed of sulphur-containing compounds: allicin, diallyl disulfide, diallyl trisulfide and others.

Garlic was used for the treatment of amoebic dysentery by Albert Schweizer in Africa and its antibiotic activity was first noted by Louis Pasteur. Garlic's antiseptic action was used in the prevention of gangrene during the first and second world wars. Herbalists are now using garlic in combination with other herbs or by itself in the treatment of the common cold, sinusitis, and upper respiratory tract infections and it is mentioned in the *British Herbal Pharmacopoeia* for the treatment of these conditions.

The very pungent odour in garlic investigations have shown it is allicin. Research shows that allicin could be the major active constituent in garlic that inhibits the growth of staphylococcus, streptococcus, bacillus, *Brucella* and *Vibrio* species at low concentrations. This would suggest that deodorised garlic may not be as efficacious.

Garlic also has anti-viral effects. Garlic was shown to protect mice infected with influenza virus from infection. It also enhanced the neutralising anti-body production when given with influenza vaccine.

Many studies have been carried out demonstrating garlic's effect on influenza B, herpes simplex, coxsackie viruses, rhinovirus and *Candida albicans.*

The second herb is *Echinacea. Echinacea's* use as an anti-viral and immune stimulating herb is well documented. The extracts from the root of the purple coneflower possess an interferon-like action. This is probably because of its polysaccharide components. These polysaccharides bind themselves to the activated carbohydrate receptors of the T-lymphocytes. This action results in the production of interferon and enhances T-cell mitogenesis, phagocytosis and increased natural killer cell activity.

This activity in vivo results in T-cell transformation. This transformation enhances cytotoxic killing of viruses. The release of interferons, as previously mentioned, also have the ability to block the transcription of viral RiboNucleic Acid (RNA) by the synthesis of intracellular proteins.

The result of this action leads to destruction of the invading virus and an increase in the number of T-lymphocytes making *Echinacea* an ideal herb to consider for diseases such as influenza and post-viral syndrome.

Vitamin C is used by most people looking for a natural way of treating the common cold. The reason for their choice was based on the work carried out by Professor Linus Pauling. Many people have said that Linus Pauling's work has not been vindicated in recent trials. However, I do not believe this to be true. Recent double-blind trials on vitamin C have shown that the symptoms of the common cold can be dramatically reduced by the taking of 2000 mg of vitamin C daily. It is probable that ascorbic acid assists the immune system and acts against pathogens, especially bacteria and viruses.

Vitamin C levels of white blood cells have been shown to decrease with depressed immunological function. Viral infection rapidly depletes leucocyte ascorbate and varying degrees of non-specific immunosuppression are now recognised to accompany such infections.

At my Clinic using a combination containing garlic, echinacea, beta-carotene and vitamin E, vitamin C in the treatment of many viral and virus related illnesses has shown successful results. The most common would be patients presenting with influenza or common colds and although full double-blind trials have not been carried out, patient trials have demonstrated dramatic improvement.

I have also used this combination of herbs and nutrients when treating patients suffering from post-viral syndrome and those who are constantly contracting viral infections. The results of these patient studies have shown a marked improvement in the patients' resistance to infection.

St John's Wort

Recent research studies have shown that the herb St John's Wort demonstrated anti AIDS activity. Laboratory experiments at New York University and at the Weizmann Institute of Science in Israel demonstrated that two compounds from St John's Wort inhibit a variety of retroviruses.

Other studies have shown that hypericin and psuedohypericin, the actives isolated from St John's Wort, showed potent antiviral activity including anti-human immunodeficiency virus. These results were reported in *Biochemical and Biophysical Research Communications* 185 (3), 1989.

Although more research needs to be carried out, the results so far are promising and St John's Wort in combination with antioxidants, could be the answer to AIDS and multiple sclerosis, a retro-viral condition comparable to AIDS.

SUPPLEMENTS:

St John's Wort	follow directions on bottle
Echinacea	500 mg dired herb twice daily
vitamin C	6000 mg daily
Bio ACE	(anti-oxidant formula)
garlic	2000 mg equivalent to fresh herb
evening primrose oil	1 capsule 3 times daily
cod liver oil	5ml daily
multi-mineral	1 daily

IMPOTENCY

Ginseng, in combination with sarsaparilla and serenoa, could be useful for males over 40 years of age to help increase sexual rejuvenation and vitality and is useful in the treatment of non-malignant prostatic enlargement.

An interesting study was carried out on ginseng by Professor Lakhovsky who said that ginseng emits an ultra-violet type of mitogenetic or gurwitch radiation also given off by the human body. Once ingested, these radiations increase the vital activity of the cells and organs they come in contact with.

Ginseng has also been used for the treatment of reproductive problems in men. Studies have shown ginseng promotes growth of the testes and increases spermatogenesis in rabbits. It could therefore be useful as a supplement for impotence.

SUPPLEMENTS

ginseng	100 mg twice daily
200 mg dried herb	three times daily
Bio Zinc	1 tablet daily
vitamin E	500 IU daily
Naturetime Multi	
Vitamin Mineral	1 tablet daily

NOTE: Ginseng should not be taken in large amounts over long periods.

INDIGESTION OR DYSPEPSIA

Indigestion (or dyspepsia) is not a specific ailment as the symptoms can be due to gastro-intestinal disorders of various kinds.

Often the body's outcry is because of an unhealthy lifestyle. It is often caused by eating more than you really need to survive; eating food too quickly, which could be a sign of anxiety or stress; swallowing air when you eat; improper chewing, often associated with poor teeth, dentures, too much fat in the diet; constipation. All of these problems can bring about indigestion leading to symptoms such as nausea, just not feeling right, headaches, weakness, flatulence, heartburn, disease.

Indigestion takes away the joy of living and it can be quite debilitating, leaving people lethargic and uncomfortable.

The first thing is to look at dividing one's daily intake into three or four well-spaced, nutritiously-balanced meals containing plenty of roughage, raw fresh fruits and vegetables and the proper distribution of carbohydrates, protein and fats.

Take time out to enjoy the meal. Plan meals so that they are not rushed. An example of rushing your food is when you eat a hamburger while driving the car or when you rush down a meal in 10 or 15 minutes. This doesn't allow the digestive juices and enzymes to work and proper mastication of the food is lost, resulting in indigestion, incorrect absorption and the feeling of lassitude and ill-health.

There are some herbs which can help. *Lactobacillus acidophilus* plus pectin can be helpful in balancing out the natural gut flora which can often be upset following a course of antibiotics or intestinal diseases. It also helps digest food. Slippery elm is good as it has soothing and antacid properties, settling the stomach and healing any ulcers that can occur with indigestion. For excessive flatulence add charcoal to the diet. One tablet 3 times daily when suffering. It can also be used with animals.

SUPPLEMENTS

Digestive Aid (contains slippery elm and natural enzymes)	1 tablet 3 times daily
lactobacillus acidophilus	1 capsule containing 2.5 billion bacilli daily
goldenseal	follow directions
peppermint	drink 3 to 4 cups of peppermint tea daily or take 0.2 ml daily of peppermint oil
sodium sulphate (celloid)	200 mg twice daily
magnesium phosphate (celloid)	200 mg twice daily

INSOMNIA

Insomnia is a common condition that affects almost one-third of the population. The causes of insomnia include biochemical imbalances and psychological problems. Biochemical imbalances can be treated by diet and natural remedies.

We need sleep for our nervous system to function properly. If we are deprived of sleep for long periods, we may suffer from irritability, hallucinations and delusions.

There are four stages of sleep.

Stage 1 is the lightest stage of sleep. There is slow eye rolling, some muscle twitching and a drop in body temperature.

Stage 2 sleep deepens slightly. EEG (electroencephalograph) measurement shows some bursts of activity.

Stage 3 This is a much deeper sleep. The EEG now slows to a larger wave pattern.

Stage 4 occurs about 40 minutes after falling asleep. This is our lowest ebb. The EEG pattern is now a slow wave. We stay in this pattern for approximately 40 minutes. It is also at this stage that bed-wetting can occur in children. Just before the very deep sleep of *Stage 4*, it is possible to be easily awakened. Many people then have difficulty in falling back to sleep if awakened at this stage.

We now return to a new Stage 1. This is called REM (Rapid-Eye-Movement) sleep. Our breathing becomes irregular and our eyes move quickly from side to side although still closed. This is our dreaming phase. If people don't achieve the REM phase, they can awake still feeling a need for sleep. This is also a phase where the slightest sound can wake the light sleeper. This pattern continues 4 to 5 times a night concluding with our awakening.

Exercise, dietary adjustments and the addition of herbs can help many poor sleepers achieve this normal sleep pattern resulting in a more mentally alert, rested and active person.

Dietary changes can help insomniacs.

Serotonin, the natural sleep-producing hormone is converted from the amino acid L-tryptophan with the aid of vitamin B6. L-tryptophan is also converted into vitamin B3. So that L-tryptophan (a natural occuring amino acid found in protein foods such as milk) is converted with the aid of vitamin B6 to serotonin and not vitamin B3, we need to include extra B3 and B6 vitamins in our diet ensuring this conversion.

To ensure adequate intake of dietary L-tryptophan, it is advisable to have a warm drink such as skim milk or soy milk — both are sources of dietary tryptophan. To ensure adequate absorption of tryptophan into the brain, it is also recommended that protein is minimised in the evening meal, and instead carbohydrates are the main component of the meal.

SUPPLEMENTS

valerian	600 mg dried herb
scullcap	300 mg dried herb
passion flower	
(*Passiflora*)	500 mg dried herb
hops	200 mg dried herb
vitamin B3	100 mg
vitamin B6	20 mg

Take the above 1 hour before bed with glass of warm low fat milk. Do not eat a large meal just before bedtime.

LEG PAIN

Intermittent Claudication

This is a problem that affects both men and women, elderly men seem to suffer from this condition more than women.

The symptoms of this condition are usually pain in the calf muscle when walking. This pain can come on slowly or it may strike suddenly. The pain is burning and cramp-like and eventually becomes so bad that the walker must stop and rest.

Intermittent claudication is caused by restricted circulation brought about by hardening and narrowing of the arteries in the legs. This reduces the blood flow and oxygen to the muscles. With the increased demand for this blood to muscles when walking and the inability of these vessels to supply it, pain and lameness soon follows.

There are many causes of the degeneration of arteries. High cholesterol causes plaque to build up in the arteries, Buerger's disease and cigarette smoking can all cause a reduction in blood flow to the legs. It is important if intermittent claudication is a problem to exercise regularly, maintain correct weight for height and if smoking to stop. Smoking causes narrowing of the arteries.

Vitamin E is by far the best treatment. Vitamin E lowers the viscosity (thins the blood), has an anti-clotting action and improves oxygen supply to the oxygen-starved tissues.

Drs Evan and Wilfrid Shute have found that alpha tocopherol vitamin E has given phenomenal success when used for the treatment of intermittent claudication.

I have found that many patients of mine have benefited and indeed their symptoms of intermittent claudication have completely gone when treated with the following supplements:

SUPPLEMENTS

vitamin E	up to 1000 IU daily

Start with 100 IU and increase slowly if suffering from high blood pressure

magnesium compound (celloid formula)	1 tablet 3 times daily
Bio C (contains bioflavonoids and vitamin C)	1 tablet daily
evening primrose oil	500 mg 1 capsule morning and night

LEG ULCERS (see Bed Sores)
LIVER HEALTH

The liver is the largest organ in the body and it performs more functions than any other organ. It produces and stores glycogen, which it synthesises from glucose. This is needed by the muscles for energy. The liver also manufactures bile which is used in the digestion of fats. It is one of the body's major detoxifiers, transforming substances that are taken into the blood by way of our intestines. The liver also synthesises prothrombin and fibrinogen which are clotting agents, and is a valuable storing house for vitamins A, D, E and K.

There are many diseases which can severely affect the liver. Abuse with certain drugs such as alcohol can cause cirrhosis of the liver which will lead to death if not treated in the early stages.

Hepatitis is a disease which inflames the liver. There are varieties of the virus: hepatitis A or infectious hepatitis, hepatitis B, or serum hepatitis and the new hepatitis C. Hepatitis infects 25% of our indigenous population. The virus can be caught through exchange of blood, saliva, or eating infected food. Clean toilet habits and washing of hands afterwards is necessary for prevention.

Certain herbs, such as dandelion and milk thistle, act as cholagogues, helping maintain a healthy liver. It also must be remembered that if the liver is not functioning properly then toxins will manifest themselves elsewhere in the body. Quite often skin disorders such as dermatitis and acne, can be directly related to a poorly functioning liver.

Most blood-cleaning herbs *per se*, act on the organs that eliminate toxins from the body and help them in their job. Dandelion has been said to have the ability to dissolve gallstones and combines well with blueberry for use in the treatment of cholecystitis (inflammation of the gallbladder), jaundice and gallstones. Three cups of dandelion coffee daily will help maintain a healthy liver. Another herb used for liver disease is boldo.

Zinc helps the liver release the storage of vitamin A. The B group of vitamins is also important for a healthy liver. Again, correct nutrition so that you eat a balanced diet, control weight and abstain from alcohol and toxic drugs such as paracetamol, which can affect the liver.

SUPPLEMENTS

Milk thistle	1ml of 1:1 fluid extract 3 times daily
dandelion tea	3 cups daily
Bio Zinc	1 tablet daily

Sustained Release
  Multi B Vitamin
  Formula   1 tablet daily
sodium sulphate 200 mg 1 tablet three times daily
A herbal complex containing blueberry, boldo and dandelion will
help maintain proper liver function.

MEDICATION AND DRUGS (see Prescribed Drugs)

MEMORY

Some medications, such as anti-anxiety medications can cause
memory loss. Quite often our short term memory does not seem
to be as good as it used to be. We forget little things. We always
remember the name of our mother and events in the past but
little items seem to be forgotten, new facts and dates go astray.

To maintain a functioning memory it is very important to have
a well-balanced diet with a variety of foods daily. There are
vitamins and minerals in these foods that are essential for correct function of the nervous system. We need to activate our
brains, reading and recalling past events. Getting memory working is very important. We should not stagnate especially as we
age. We must keep our minds active.

One herb is *ginkgo.* Herbs can help the memory. One of the
oldest tree species in the world. *Ginkgo* improves cerebral circulation (blood flow to the brain) at the same time increasing the
brain's intake of carbohydrate. Ginkgo has proven to be of particular value for the treatment of short-term memory loss.

There are many other nutrients of benefit in improving
memory and/or slowing-down the onset of senile dementia. They
include lecithin and multivitamins. A number of trials have show
that supplementation may be beneficial in retarding Alzheimer's
disease. *Panax ginseng* can also be helpful, and also in combination with *ginkgo.*

SUPPLEMENTS

Ginseng   100 mg daily
multivitamin formula   1 daily
lecithin   2000 mg daily

vitamin E   500 IU daily
Gingko plus formula   3 times daily
Do not use aluminium cookware or deodorant containing aluminium as high aluminium levels in the blood have been reported
in adults with memory loss.

MENOPAUSE (change of life)

Menopause or the cessation of the menstrual cycle, occurs in
women usually between the age of 38 and 58 years. It is the
result of the loss of the menses and is a natural occurrence that
affects all women. Menopausal symptoms may also follow a hys-
terectomy. Symptoms of menopause can come on suddenly or
over a period of time. Usually menstruation stops slowly decreas-
ing a little each month or they may stop for a few months and
then start again. These symptoms may only last a few months or
may continue for up to five years. There is no absolute.

The onset of change of life may in some women be *signalled* by
hot flushes, headache, arthritic pain, palpitations, depression and
emotional instability. In others, the symptoms, apart from the
cessation of the menstrual cycle, may not be noticeable.

Menopause is not the end of womanhood or sexuality. For
some, the opposite is the rule. Menopause is only the end of the
reproductive cycle, it is not a sign of old age. This change had
nothing to do with greying of the hair or a loss of sexual desire;
post-menopausal women can live a very enjoyable and active life
in all respects.

If you are going through menopause and the symptoms are
intense then natural therapy has a lot to offer, before you consider the alternative of oestrogen treatment. A number of studies
have shown that vitamin E supplementation can eliminate or
reduce the symptoms associated with menopause, particularly
hot flushes.

Dong quai has been used in Asia for thousands of years and its
reputation is second only to ginseng. Dong quai is regarded as
the "female remedy" and has been used successfully for the
treatment of many female disorders including menopause,
amenorrhea and dysmenorrhea.

Dong quai contains phytoestrogens (plant oestrogens). These
natural plant oestrogens compete with the oestrogen in the body
for binding sites. The phytoestrogens in Dong quai produce
oestrogenic activity when the body's oestrogen levels are low as is

the case in menopause. The ability of the phytoestrogens to occupy oestrogen receptor sites also helps high oestrogen levels. Dong quai is specifically of use for the treatment of menopausal hot flushes. Evening primrose oil in conjunction with herbs and vitamins for the treatment of many hormonal disorders including menopause has met with good results.

Oats are of value when used for the treatment of menopausal depression and neurasthenia. Avena stimulates both the motor and sensory systems. This stimulation gives a lift and elevation in mood.

SUPPLEMENTS

Dong quai	500 mg 3 times daily
oats	1000 mg 3 times daily
vitamin E	500 IU daily
Executive B Complex (stress B group formula)	1 tablet daily
evening primrose oil	500 mg 1 capsule 3 times daily

MENSTRUATION

Primary dysmenorrhea or painful menstruation affects about half the female population in Australia, the symptoms include mild to severe pains (cramps) in the abdomen, lower back and in the legs. They may also be accompanied by heavy or scant bleeding.

The causes could be a number of things ranging from anxiety, lack of exercise, hormone imbalance, constipation, pelvic inflammation, or endometritis. What ever the cause, dysmenorrhea can cause a reduction in the quality of life.

Eat foods that are high in fibre as this will help eliminate constipation. Water is also important and you must drink between 6 to 8 glasses of pure water each day.

Vitamin E has been show to help relieve the pain and help normalise periods. 68% of women given vitamin E supplementation showed improvement compared to controls in an experimental placebo-controlled study.

Iron supplement may also be of benefit. When iron-deficient patients were given an iron supplement they showed marked improvement. The B group of vitamins with the mineral magnesium have also given good results.

Blueberry acts as a smooth muscle relaxant and clinical research has shown that this herb can be of value in the treatment of painful periods. Beth Root saponins are likely to interact with female hormones. This action could contribute to its ability to correct hormonal imbalances.

American Cranesbill has strong astringent properties and can help manage heavy periods in women who lack exercise.

Dong quai (*Angelica sinensis*) has been used in Asia for thousands of years and its reputation is second only to ginseng. Dong quai is regarded as the "female remedy" and has been used successfully for the treatment of many female disorders including menopause, amenorrhea and dysmenorrhea.

Dong quai contains phytoestrogens (plant oestrogens) which compete with the oestrogen in the body for binding sites. The ability of the phytoestrogens to occupy oestrogen receptor sites also help in conditions of high oestrogen levels as may be the case in dysmenorrhea.

Essential fatty acids found in fish oil and evening primrose oil have also shown to be of benefit as their action is on the prostaglanden E series that are said to produce myometrial relaxation.

SUPPLEMENTS

dong quai	500 mg 3 times daily or ginseng 100 mg twice daily
American cranesbill	500 mg 3 times daily
beth root	750 mg 3 times daily
blueberry	fresh berries daily
vitamin E	500 mg daily
PMT formula (Blackmores)	1 tablet daily
evening primrose oil	500 mg 1 capsule morning and night

MIGRAINE

Migraine, a word derived from Greek, means half a head. This often describes a headache that attacks only one side of the head. This usually starts with interference to vision in one eye, seeing zig-zag patterns, shooting lights, or having blindspots. Pain, accompanied by nausea, blurred vision, tingling and numbness in the limbs, may last for up to 18 hours. Migraines are often hereditary and most sufferers are women. Sufferers have abnormal levels of certain brain chemicals that often cause dilation and contraction of blood vessels.

Allergies are a common cause of migraine and migraine headaches may also be caused by liver malfunction. It is a good idea to avoid salt, and acid-producing food such as meat, cereal, bread and grains. Fried and greasy foods should also be avoided. Hot dogs, luncheon meats, monosodium glutamate, oranges, dairy products, especially hard cheese, and chocolate, have also been attributed with precipitating migraine attacks.

One should look at a raw, natural food diet, similar to that of a hypoglycaemic diet, staying away from processed and refined carbohydrates. The vitaimin B group has shown to be advantageous to many people suffering from migraine and up to 1000 mg of vitamin C should also be considered.

Once a migraine strikes, it is very difficult to alleviate the pain. The answer lies in prevention. Modern medical studies show that the ancient herb feverfew could be the answer. Feverfew has a long history in treating various aches and pains, arthritis, high blood pressure, skin conditions, fevers, inflammation and headaches.

Modern studies have confirmed its benefits with particular regard to its use as a preventative for migraine headaches. This was convincingly demonstrated by a definitive double-blind study conducted in England in 1985, using capsules of freeze-dried feverfew powder at a dosage level of 50 mg per day. Results indicated a significant protection against migraine attacks in those patients taking the capsules. Other clinical studies have backed up this finding, even with patients who had failed to respond to orthodox medical treatment.

There is only one variety of feverfew which produces this result. This is *Tanacetum parthenium* (the synonym is *Chrysanthemum parthenium*). Only this species ensures the highest concentration of active herbal constituents. According to authorities, feverfew quality depends on optimum harvest time and the part of the plant picked. The product should be derived from *leaf* before budding, to retain maximum potency. The leaf has an extremely bitter taste, which is overcome by taking the herb in capsule form.

The efficacy of feverfew is now proven and may be one of the best measures against migraine headache. It is important we understand that feverfew is *not* a pain-relieving herb and will not help you once your headache has begun.

SUPPLEMENTS

feverfew
   (standardised extract)   50 mg each morning

MOUTH ULCERS

Mouth ulcers can be very painful, and can be triggered by food allergies. Pineapples can cause mouth ulcers in sensitive people. Little pimples on the tongue, or bites on the inside of cheeks, can ulcerate. These can be very painful and need to be addressed.

You can mix up a little formula at home to dab on these ulcers. Mix one third glycerine, one third oil of cloves and one third tea-tree oil, together, dab onto a cotton bud and apply to the mouth ulcers. You will find they heal very quickly. The oil of cloves helps numb the pain. Add zinc and the B group of vitamins to your diet to help prevent them occurring.

SUPPLEMENTS

vitamin B complex   1 tablet morning and night
zinc   25 mg daily

MULTIPLE SCLEROSIS (see Immune System)

NIGHT VISION AND EYESIGHT

Beta-carotene is the natural yellow colouring found in vegetables. It was in the news during the Second World War when it was said that pilots in the British Airforce were fed carrots as a source of nutrient to improve their night vision. Many people believed that this was how they could spot the invading bombers but the truth was that the British had invented radar first which the Germans had not as yet discovered.

Recent evidence does show that beta-carotene and vitamin A are very important nutrients for the production of visual purple and this visual purple in our eyes is needed for night vision. Therefore, a diet rich in foods containing beta-carotene and vitamin A is required for us to have normal night vision. Without these nutrients we are unable to re-manufacture our visual purple after it has been damaged. Some of the things that can damage visual purple and reduce night vision are television screens, VDU screens, and bright lights.

Blueberry, helps improve night vision. Taking the extract of the herb also restores visual acuity after exposure to bright light (glare) and can improve vision in low light.

We should be looking at a natural supplement of beta-carotene if we are not getting enough in our diets from leafy green and yellow vegetables. Beta-carotene is also an antioxidant. (For more information on antioxidants, refer to antioxidants in this book.)

SUPPLEMENTS

natural beta-carotene (provitamin A)	6mg daily with main meal
antioxidants, vitamin A, C and E	vitamin A 10000 daily vitamin C 1000 mg daily vitamin E 500 daily
blueberry	100 mg extract 3 times daily

OSTEOARTHRITIS (also see Arthritis)

Degenerative joint disease (osteoarthritis) can affect anyone although menopausal women are most vulnerable.

This is a mild and degenerative joint disease mainly affecting the weight-bearing joints but it can also affect the spine and neck. Weight reduction is very important in order to lessen stress on the joints.

Hot and cold water treatment of the joints can also help, four minutes in hot water, followed by one minute in cold water several times daily 15 to 20 minutes at a time. Be careful not to damage skin tissue with the hot water.

Walking and swimming are good exercise and must be carried out daily for 15 to 30 minutes. This will help reduce pain, increase mobility, and decrease rate of bone loss.

Use the same diet as that used for Crystal Arthritis.

SUPPLEMENTS

Same as rheumatoid arthritis

OSTEOPOROSIS

Women are more affected by this disease than men. They have a lighter bone structure and the changes in their hormonal pattern after menopause seems to accelerate this disease.

Osteoporosis is a leaching of calcium from the bones that begins around 30 years of age. You really have to make sure that you are getting enough calcium in your diet: 800–1200 mg of calcium phosphate per day is required. If you are not receiving this amount, then you run the risk of osteoporosis when you grow older.

Foods containing calcium, such as dairy products and fish, are very important sources and should be included in the diet or supplementation.

Exercising regularly is recommended as this also prevents bone loss. The best forms are swimming and walking each day, so, after a hard day's work, before sitting down in front of the television, take the dog for a walk. With exercise you can increase the size and strength of your bones.

The diet should contain foods with a high alkaline ash residue, such as vegetables and fruits. Recent evidence published in the *Journal of American Geriatrics* in 1982 showed that meat and other high protein foods, most cereal grains and starches with a high acid ash residue, increase calcium excretion and bone loss. Increase dairy products and green leafy vegetables and decrease protein in your diet.

Avoid coffee. Studies have shown that urinary calcium excretion increases significantly after ingestion of caffeine contained in coffee. Smokers often have an earlier menopause than non-smokers and menopause speeds up osteoporosis. Alcohol may also reduce bone mass.

SUPPLEMENTS

calcium phosphate	2000 mg daily
vitamin D	400 mg daily
folic acid	5 mg daily
magnesium compound	3 tablets daily
Multivitamin mineral (sustained release)	1 tablet daily

PAINFUL MENSTRUATION (See Menstruation)

PRE-MENSTRUAL TENSION (PMT)

Pre-menstrual tension affects 70% of women. Symptoms include depression, headaches, painful breasts, water retention, fatigue. Actually, it should be called pre-menstrual syndrome. The tension side is only part of the problem.

PMT can be divided into four subgroups: PMT A (anxiety), PMT C (craving), PMT D (depression) and PMT H (hyperhydration).

Some vitamins and herbs can be of great value and give positive results when used for treatment of PMT. One of the vitamins is vitamin B6. Vitamin B6 acts as a mild diuretic and has proven to be of enormous value to women who suffer pre-menstrual tension. Include it with a multivitamin formula so that you are not just taking one vitamin by itself. A PMT formula available in health food stores has been adjusted to suit all requirements.

If you are showing signs of fluid retention such as painful breasts or swollen fingers, then you should supplement your diet with celery, dandelion, and juniper tablets. These are natural herbal diuretics and can relieve the symptoms of painful breasts and fluid retention. Evening primrose oil has been clinically proven to decrease the symptoms of PMT. *Glycyrrhiza* is a recommended supplement as it competes with aldosterone for binding sites. Aldosterone, a hormone secreted by the adrenal cortex, is elevated in the blood 7 days before menstruation.

Limit coffee and dairy products and eat vegetable protein.

SUPPLEMENTS

vitamin B6	100 mg daily
vitamin B1	100 mg daily
PMT multivitamin formula	1 tablet or capsule daily
evening primrose oil	500 mg 1 three times daily
magnesium phosphate	200 mg twice daily
liquorice	500 mg daily for 5 days before menstruation

PREGNANCY

Pregnancy and child birth is a special part of a woman's life. This joyous event is the creation of a new life and the start of years of joy, worry, happiness, and anxiety.

Having a healthy pregnancy is the first and most important step in your new baby's life. It is a great responsibility on both the expectant mother and the father. Their lifestyle and the nutrition of the mother will play the most important part in the development of the unborn baby.

Many studies have shown that a lack of some vitamins and minerals in the diet could be associated with some types of birth defects and that supplements may prevent these defects occurring. The birth defects that may be prevented by taking a multivitamin supplement before and during the pregnancy include spina bifida and harelip.

Correct eating habits, a balanced diet, and supplements of a multivitamin mineral formula could help prevent many of the problems that may be associated with pregnancy and birth defects.

The expectant mother should not drink alcohol. Studies have shown that even mild alcohol ingestion during pregnancy may result in hyperactivity, short attention span, and emotional problems in the resulting children. Alcohol can also cause other deformities in the unborn baby. Alcohol foetal syndrome is one and is thought to be caused by the mother consuming alcohol during the first 3 months of pregnancy.

Drugs and smoking can also cause many problems to both mother and the foetus. Your medical practitioner or naturopath should be consulted before taking any medication. They will advise you as to their safety. All confinements should be under the care of a medical specialist.

Scientific clinical studies have shown that supplements of vitamin E may be effective in preventing habitual abortion (miscarriage). Foods that are high in vitamin E such as wheat germ, whole grains and cold pressed vegetable oils should be included in the diet.

Solanine is a toxin found in green potatoes. This chemical has been shown to cause miscarriages. It is important therefore not to eat new potatoes or potatoes with any green spots if pregnant.

Exercise is an important part of everybody's lifestyle and especially for the expectant mother. Exercise tones the muscles, improves circulation, helps control weight and can make delivery easier. There are many ante-natal classes run by most hospitals. The trained nursing staff who give these classes will advise the correct exercise program for you.

Some evidence states that vitamin B6 (pyridoxine) may help relieve the symptons of morning sickness. These include nausea and vomiting. Usually the amount of vitamin B6 contained in a good multi-vitamin formula is sufficient. However, high doses of B6 should be avoided late in the pregnancy as studies have shown that high dose vitamin B6 may shut off breast milk. It must therefore be reduced before delivery in nursing mothers.

I have found that peppermint tea is helpful in relieving the symptoms of morning sickness as can taking ginger. Drink one cup of peppermint tea and eat a piece of toast before getting out of bed in the morning. This will need the help of the father-to-be and he should remember that his duties start at conception.

SUPPLEMENTS

folic acid	0.8 mg daily during pregnancy. (folic acid requirement doubles during pregnancy)
calcium	1000 mg to 1500 mg daily, 2000 mg daily during lactation (calcium requirements double during pregnancy)
magnesium	500 mg daily
iron phosphate	15 mg 3 times daily
Naturetime Multivitamin Mineral (sustained release)	1 tablet daily
evening primrose oil	500 mg 1 capsule morning and night (supplement may be beneficial during pregnancy-induced hypertension)
For morning sickness travel calm ginger	1 tablet 3 times daily
peppermint tea	1 cup in morning before getting out of bed and then 1 cup 3 times daily
red raspberry leaf tea	Drink 3 cups a day during the third trimester. Red raspberry leaf tea has been traditionally used as a uterine tonic and to help relieve the pain of childbirth.

PRESCRIBED DRUGS

Taking prescribed medications with most vitamins is safe as is taking herbal complexes that are available through health food stores. However, you should always check with your doctor, your pharmacist or your naturopath. They are all trained to know what can go with what.

An example would be Warfarin. Warfarin is used to thin the blood (anticoagulant). This medication should not be taken with any other substance that has anticoagulant properties, for example, *ginkgo*, aspirin and high dose vitamin E, without the advice of your medical practitioner.

The contraceptive pill for instance destroys vitamin B6. We know that certain antibiotics can destroy the B group and can also have an effect on the intestinal gut flora, diminishing the bacteria which is very important for processing vitamin B and manufacturing antibodies. So really, vitamins can be destroyed by medications but usually, the medication is not affected by vitamins.

Some foods should not be taken with medications. Certain antibiotics, such as tetracyclins, if taken with a protein such as milk, can bind to that protein and make itself ineffective. Check with your medical practitioner.

PROSTATE PROBLEMS

For the treatment of benign prostatic enlargement there are two herbs that can be very helpful.

The herb saw palmetto (*Serenoa repens*) should be used. Serenoa acts in toning the male reproductive system, particularly the prostate and can reduce prostatic hypertrophy.

Horsetail acts as a strong diuretic and is of benefit when used for urinary and prostatic diseases. Horsetail has been used in the treatment of irritable symptoms of the urinary system. It stimulates the bladder and kidneys and helps move any stones. Zinc is also needed as many studies show that a lack of zinc in the diet could be associated with prostatic enlargement.

SUPPLEMENTS

Serenoa	750 mg twice daily
horsetail	1700 mg twice daily
zinc	25 mg twice daily
antioxidant formula	1 tablet twice daily

PSORIASIS (see Skin Disorders)

RAYNAUD'S SYNDROME (see Cold Hands and Feet)

RHEUMATOID ARTHRITIS (see Arthritis)

RINGING IN THE EARS (see Tinnitus)

SINUSITIS

Sinusitis is inflammation of the sinuses or passages which are found in the bones surrounding the nose and eyes.

Sinusitis is a debilitating problem that can cause pain, mild fever, headaches, stuffy nose and depression. Allergies are a common cause (see 'Allergies'). Dairy products can be a problem and should be avoided. There are some herbs that can help relieve the problem. Horseradish is one. Horseradish forms mustard oil in the body and it gives off mustard gas. This can help clear out the sinuses. Garlic is another herb that can help. It has anti-bacterial activity and will help dry up the infected sinuses.

Elder flower (*Sambucus nigra*) is a herb that I have found very helpful when used for the treatment of sinus problems, especially when used in conjunction with *Echinacea*, garlic, and horseradish.

Vitamin A supplementation is also beneficial as it strengthens the mucous membranes in the nose and throat. The anti-inflammatory properties of the essential fatty acids found in cod liver oil give relief from the inflammation and pain.

SUPPLEMENTS

elder flower	1250 mg twice daily
eyebright	1000 mg twice daily
horseradish	300 mg twice daily
garlic	2000 mg fresh herb twice daily
liquorice	200 mg twice daily

Echinacea	375 mg twice daily
cod liver oil	5 ml daily
vitamin C	2000 mg daily
iron phosphate	15 mg 3 times daily
potassium chloride	32 mg 3 times daily

SKIN DISORDERS

Skin disorders are quite debilitating to many people because they often affect the face and hands and can be unsightly and very embarrassing. Probably the most common skin disorders are atopic eczema and eczema dermatitis. Eczema, is inflammation of the skin which often occurs when there is an irritant. The sufferer is easily upset and of nervous temperament, and often has a dry, scaly skin. Eczema usually affects the knees, face, neck and elbows. It is a dull, red, scaly patch that can become extremely itchy. In most medical treatment steroid ointments are used which have short term effects and dramatic side effects. The naturophathic approach involves the patient avoiding allergens and controlling or avoiding stressful situations.

Contact eczema such as housewives' eczema, where detergents cause a flare up on the hands, is the most common. Occupational eczema from contact with acids, alkalines, and allergens, is important to detect. If this is not the source then look at the diet. Vitamin A and zinc and the herbs sarsparilla, red clover, burdock, and dandelion can help neutralise the problems that are causing eczema. Evening primrose oil taken in large doses has proven effective in scientific studies when used for the treatment of many skin disorders. Ointments containing chickweed, pine coal tar, and juniper berry can also help reduce inflammation, stop itching, and speed up the healing process.

SUPPLEMENTS

evening primrose oil	500 mg 2 capsules 3 times daily
bio zinc	1 tablet morning and night
sarsparilla complex	1 table 3 times daily
cod liver oil	5 ml daily
multivitamin mineral (sustained release)	1 tablet each morning
External treatment:	
chick weed compound	
Eczema balm	
Dermatone	

SMOKING (see Cigarette Smoking)

SORE THROAT

When you have a sore throat it can affect your everyday life. Every time you want to speak it seems to get worse. It is hard to swallow, especially in the mornings, where you are dehydrated.

One of the old remedies used was two drops of eucalyptus in a teaspoon of honey. This is very effective, but first you need to remove the phlegm and mucus. Phlegm and mucus gather in the throat and can cause irritation. It is also an ideal medium for bacteria to breed in. A good way to get rid of it is to gargle with warm water and salt. Dissolve a couple of teaspoons of salt in warm water, gargle and then spit it out. This will soothe the throat and remove the mucus. Salt is also a very good antiseptic that can kill bacteria on the mucus membrane of the mouth and throat.

The herb slippery elm is very soothing. If you suck on slippery elm tablets, the mucilage in the herb coats the throat, helping reduce inflammation and pain.

Iron phosphate, potassium chloride and zinc are minerals that also have anti-inflammatory properties. These can be found in cold tablet formulas. Usually a sore throat is the sign of more to come. If this is not treated promptly, further upper respiratory infections or the common cold or flu may follow so help build up your resistance by taking the supplements.

SUPPLEMENTS

cold tablets containing iron phosphate and potassium chloride	1 tablet 3 times daily
slippery elm	suck 1 tablet 3 times daily
vitamin C	2000 mg daily
Echinacea	as directed on bottle (extract or dried herb)
garlic	2000 mg dried herb-enteric coated daily

STRAINS AND SPRAINS

Many people rub a sprain or strain immediately with a heat rub or with hot and cold compresses. This is wrong. Apply cold water or ice to the area as soon as possible. This should be done at 20-minute intervals for the first half day to stop the swelling and to help reduce the injury and bruising. This is very important. We need to start the healing process and this can be done by rubbing on a cream containing comfrey. Comfrey ointment speeds up the healing process. On the second day, start using heat rubs to return circulation and speed up the healing process. Remember, ice first and heat the next day.

The sprain should be supported using an elastic or conforming bandage. It may be walked on if there is no pain. A little discomfort is alright. Rest the sprained joint as much as possible by elevating it above the heart. This will help reduce pain and swelling.

SUPPLEMENTS

vitamin C	2000 mg daily
zinc	25 mg daily
silica	25 mg daily
cod liver oil	5 ml daily

Localised treatment:
Comfrey ointment and a heat rub.

STRESS

Stress affects everyone at some time. Stress can be mild. Everyday stress people encounter paying mortgages, rent, telephone bills, driving to work, having problems with the car is associated with lifestyle and commitments. There is severe stress such as a family bereavement, or marriage break-up, or not being able to pay the rent. These types of stressful situations quite often need special attention.

The vitamin B group is of benefit as this group of vitamins is essential to help maintain proper nervous system function. Along with a well-balanced diet, a B group combined with small amounts of the anti-stress herbs, scullcap, valerian and *Passiflora* can help us survive stressful times.

Long-term stress can depress our adrenal hormones and drain us of energy. If suffering this depression-related stress, there are three herbs that can help give a lift and a return to normal life. They are oats, rosemary, and kola.

Scullcap, valerian, *Passiflora*, hops, and gentian in combination can be a very potent anti-stress formula and can really help you get through those very difficult times. They are non-habit forming and very safe. Herbalists have used them for hundreds of years.

So, don't forget, try to relax (meditation can help) and enjoy life. If you are a hard case, counselling might be appropriate; if not, try dancing, singing, or yoga classes.

SUPPLEMENTS

high potency multi B formula	1 tablet daily	
herbal formula containing		
scullcap	475 mg	The amount needed depends on
valerian	300 mg	the individual. This type of
hops	750 mg	formula is available from your
gentian		health food store.
potassium phosphate (celloid)	35 mg 3 times daily	
magnesium phosphate (celloid)	65 mg 3 times daily	

TINNITUS AND VERTIGO

A ringing in the ears, or noises in the ears is called tinnitus. Many people suffer from this problem, especially at they get older. If you are suffering from tinnitus have it properly diagnosed by your practitioner, to determine the cause. There are many causes, the main one being an interruption of the cerebral blood supply or a functional disorder, or it could be drug-related. Aspirin and quinine can cause tinnitus.

If it is a circulation problem, then *ginkgo* can help. Gingko has been used for thousands of years and is the oldest tree in the world, or one of the oldest species in the world. Many medical trials have been carried out into its uses for cerebral vascular disorders and tinnitus and for vertigo, a disturbance of the sense of balance, are two of the types of disorders which can be treated.

Other herbs that have shown to be of benefit are black cohosh and betony. The minerals magnesium phosphate and potassium phosphate have shown good results.

The diet should be a low cholesterol, low refined-carbohydrate diet. Essential omega 6 and 3 fatty acids are important as supplements which increase red-cell deformability and a reduction in blood viscosity which can improve blood flow to the affected areas.

SUPPLEMENTS

Ginkgo	400 mg 3 times daily
garlic	2000 mg equivalent to fresh herb
cod liver oil	5ml daily
magnesium phosphate	200 mg daily
potassium phosphate	100 mg daily
black cohosh	800 mg twice daily
betony	500 mg twice daily
vitamin E	500 IU daily

TRAVEL SICKNESS

Travel sickness is a problem that many of us have had to cope with especially if we have children. Children are quite often sick in the car, or in the boat, or in the plane, or any time that they are subject to motion.

When children get travel sickness or motion sickness there are quite a few things you can do and one of the most important is to keep them busy and occupied. Word games are a good idea as they have to keep looking out of the window and so they are not looking at things within the car. Reading while driving is not a good idea as it can upset their balance and cause them to be sick. Encourage them to look at the scenery and point out things as they are going along. Most effective is to put the sick child in the front seat.

Don't let them eat greasy foods and fill them up with foods that are going to make them nauseous. What you should be looking at is to give the children wholesome foods the night before and a small breakfast before travelling as it is very important that they do have something to eat and drink.

One of the things that I have used successfully is ginger. Ginger is often used in cooking, but to take ginger before you go on the trip and during the trip, can really make a difference in the prevention of motion sickness. It does not have the harsh side effects of some antihistamines and other travel-sickness medications. Ginger is gentle to the stomach, helps with flatulence, and also helps the digestive system.

SUPPLEMENTS

Travel Calm Ginger	1 tablet 2 hours before travel then 1 tablet every hour during travel.
vitamin B6	50 mg daily

VARICOSE VEINS

Varicose veins affect men and women equally.

You have to rest your legs, above your heart, by lying down and putting a pillow under your ankles, twice a day for about 20 minutes if possible. It is important not to wear clothes that are too tight, especially underclothing. This can cut off the circulation and cause a build-up of pressure in the veins, leading to breakdown in the valves which can result in varicose veins. Constipation and pregnancy can also restrict blood flow to the legs. It is therefore important to eat a well-balanced diet high in fibre and drink 6 to 8 glasses of water every day. This will help eliminate problems such as constipation.

Include vitamin E in your diet. Eat foods that contain vitamin E, such as whole wheat, grains and cold pressed vegetable oils. The wheat germ is very rich in vitamin E and will increase oxygen to the area by improving circulation. Bioflavonoids and vitamin C can be of benefit. The combination of these two nutrients prevent capillary fragility and star-like veins that may appear. Fish oil containing omega 3 fatty acids will thin the blood and also help relieve pain associated with inflammation.

Keep your weight down. Overweight increases the load on the vascular system and can worsen the problem.

SUPPLEMENTS

vitamin E	500 to 1000 IU daily (start with 100 IU)
calcium fluoride 6x	one tablet 3 times daily
Bio C (contains vitamin C and bioflavonoids)	1 tablet morning and night
zinc	25 mg elemental 1 tablet daily
fish oil	1000 mg 1 capsule 3 times daily

VERTIGO (see Tinnitus)

WARTS

Warts are caused by a virus and can be transmitted. Children usually grow out of warts but while the problem exists it must be attended to.

First of all we need to address nutrition. Make sure they have good, wholesome food and that they eat from a variety of foods every day as this is important to help build their resistance. Include a herb called *Echinacea* which is an anti-viral herb, along with garlic and onions. Vitamins A, C and E are antioxidants and therefore can help build up the immune system. These will all help to keep warts at bay.

Externally, an ointment based on the herb thuja can be applied to the wart, itself. Thuja ointment can kill the virus and the wart will fall off, even plantar warts on the feet. It is very hard to keep the ointment on so the use of a bandaid will assist.

Warts are a virus and you do recover although it may take some years. Various treatments work — burning, filing, dandelion, thistle milk. Anxiety seems to encourage them. So stick with your treatments and above all else, do not worry.

SUPPLEMENTS

	Adult dose
Echinacea	500 mg three times daily
vitamin A	10000 IU daily
vitamin C	4000 mg daily
vitamin E	500 IU daily
garlic	equivalent to 2000 mg fresh herb daily

ointment containing thuja, apply to wart three times daily.

WEIGHT LOSS

Overweight is most commonly a result of overeating and lack of exercise. Overweight and fluid retention often go together with people who have glandular problems or under-active thyroids. In such cases an iodine and phosporous deficiency may be the cause. For people who overeat, crash dieting and/or starvation dieting, can lead to major problems and if you reduce your calorie intake below 450 calories a day for any long period, you can permanently lower your metabolism, making it much harder to maintain an ideal weight.

If the calorie intake is reduced to between 1000 and 1500 calories per day, a normal healthy person will successfully reduce weight to a level where it can easily be maintained. As part of the daily dietary regime include more vegetables and fruits. Cut back on foods such as bread, cakes and excessively fatty meats and animal products. If you wish to nibble, it is good idea to keep carrots or celery in the fridge, they are not high in calories and are very satisfying.

Natural fibre tablets can be helpful and chewing one or two with a large glass of water half an hour before a meal can assist in curbing the appetite. Drinking water is also an appetite suppressant. Most of us do not drink enough water. We should be drinking 6 to 8 glasses every day. If you have a problem with fluid retention then the herbs corn silk, boldo and blueberry are very helpful. Vitamin B6 can also be of benefit. Exercise at least three times weekly for 20 minutes. This will increase your metabolism and speed up weight loss. When dieting it is a good idea to take a multivitamin mineral formula.

If you have overweight problems associated with diseases such as diabetes then you should consult your health practitioner.

WEIGHT LOSS DIET (3 weeks)

Chew two apple fibre tablets 30 minutes before each meal to help give a feeling of fullness and increases your fibre intake

BREAKFAST
100 ml of apple or grapefruit juice (unsweetened) mixed 50/50 with water

AND

1 poached egg with 1 slice of whole grain bread, lightly spread with butter.
Small serve of a wheat cereal, ¼ peach, skim milk (no sugar)

OR

slice of grilled cheese and tomato on whole-grain bread, toasted and a cup of herbal tea 30 minutes after meal

MORNING TEA
1 medium apple, orange

OR

fruit juice mixed 50/50 with water

LUNCH
2 lettuce leaves
4 cucumber slices
¼ stick celery
½ tomato
2 slices of beetroot
1 pineapple ring

OR

vegetable casserole (serves 2 people)
3 tomatoes (medium)
1 onion
150g of fresh mushroom
30g of rice
70g of celery
Boil the rice until it is half cooked and then add the other ingredients. Use a little kelp powder or other herbs to taste. Complete cooking and serve when ready.
1 baked potato small (½ potato each)
Cup of herbal tea (30 minutes after lunch)

AFTERNOON TEA
1 glass of vegetable juice

OR

1 medium apple or orange

DINNER
Grilled ¼ chicken, no skin

OR

Steamed or grilled fish or veal with lemon (100gm)
1 baked potato (in jacket)
Small serve of fruit salad for dessert (3 times per week)

AND

side salad
2 lettuce leaves
3 slices of cucumber
2 sprigs of parsley
½ pineapple ring

OR

steamed vegetables (small serve)

OR

vegetable casserole (as in lunch)

SUPPLEMENTS

Take one Naturetime multivitamin each morning with food and drink 6 to 8 glasses of water each day

HIGH FIBRE WEIGHT LOSS DIET

This is a 15-day high fibre weight loss diet. It can be used as often as required.

BREAKFAST
Half a cup of oats and add one teaspoon of unprocessed bran — with half a cup of low fat milk, half a grapefruit or half an orange (eat the whole fruit, not just the juice).

LUNCH
Tossed salad. May consist of every salad item, such as cucumber, mung bean sprouts, mushrooms, lettuce. Take these items to work and prepare fresh.

DINNER
Five ounces of fish (dry grilled or baked), chicken or turkey. Avoid all fat and skin on the poultry and eat with steamed vegetables (2 to 3 cups) of any kind.

SNACKS
Prepare carrot and cucumber sticks or celery pieces and eat whenever you are hungry. Keep them cool in the fridge — they taste great. Do not eat when you are not hungry. You may eat one piece of fruit, preferably citrus, as a snack daily.

SALAD DRESSING
Add several teaspoons to your salad.
Mix 1 cup of water to 1 cup of apple cider vinegar. Then add:
½ tsp. of basil
½ tsp. of rosemary
½ tsp. of oregano
½ tsp. of dry mustard
¼ cup of apple juice (unsweetened)
¼ cup of lemon juice
3 tsps. of parsley
1 clove of garlic (minced finely or crushed)
This flavour enhances with time — allow 12 hours.

Use only cold pressed vegetable oils such as linseed, wheatgerm, or apricot kernel oil.

FLUID
Drink 6 to 8 glasses of water daily. Avoid coffee. Drink weak tea or herbal teas with no sugar. Your total non-fat milk allowance is ½ cup daily. Alcohol will slow down your weight loss.

EXERCISE
Walk for 40 minutes or the equivalent in your chosen physical activity each day.

SUPPLEMENTS

Take one sustained release multivitamin and mineral tablet each day.

Take one kelp tablet ½ an hour before each meal with glass of water.

Chew one apple fibre tablet ½ an hour before each meal three times daily.

ZINC

Many of us wouldn't know if we are getting enough zinc in our diets or not. There are however, a couple of signs that can tell us if zinc is lacking. White spots under the fingernails, premature greying of the hair and slow healing of wounds can quite often indicate a zinc deficiency. Some evidence has indicated that stretch marks can also be caused by a lack of zinc in the diet.

Zinc is a very important mineral and constituent of many enzymes involved in digesting and burning food. It is responsible for the action of over 2000 different enzymes within the body. What we must do is include foods that are rich in zinc. Grains and nuts are probably one of the best sources. Zinc is also important for proper sexual development of young children. Recent research has shown it is important to help prevent certain prostate gland problems that may affect men as they grow older. Small signs of deficiency are hair loss, acne, aching joints, low immunity, infections which are slow to heal and fatigue.

Recent surveys carried out by the Australian Government have shown us that zinc can be deficient in many diets. According to this survey up to 80% of women in Australia could be lacking zinc in their diet. This is based on the recommended daily intake. It is very important that we look at a well-balanced diet containing fresh fruit and vegetables of different colours, meats, nuts and dairy products. The Australian soil we are growing our foods in may be lacking this very important mineral.

Supplementation may be the only way we can ensure we are receiving enough in our diets.

PART III
THE GUIDE TO HERBS
USED IN THIS BOOK

I have already talked about the value of herbs and their place in medicine to-day, for like the animals that wander this wonderful world we call earth, we are starting to realise that mother nature has given us, in the form of plants and herbs, medicine for almost all the diseases that we are afflicted with.

You only need to look at your own dog and to see an inbuilt ability, or sixth sense. If your dog is sick it will go off its food and eat grass to cleanse its system and, at the same time, it will rest until it is better. All humans have this ability to eat what is best for them and, in the past, they would eat different herbs with their meals to wade off different sicknesses. Unfortunately, we have, over thousands of years, grown further and further away from nature. Because of this, we have lost the ability to interpret our own body's needs correctly. This inability has led us further away from nature's own oldest healing medicine, herbs.

CAUTIONARY NOTE ON HERBS

Most herbs can be used safely over long periods in small amounts. However, care should be taken when using herbs that have a cumulative effect. Some of these herbs are mentioned but this book is not comprehensive and professional advise is necessary in long-term use.

Golden seal should not be taken over long periods of time because of its effect on the intestinal bacteria which can affect the absorption of Vitamin B. Lily of the valley and ephedra should not be used with persons who are suffering from a history of very high blood pressue. Comfrey and foxglove are cumulative and poisonous in large amounts.

When collecting wild herbs, know the herb that you are gathering. It is not difficult to incorrectly identify wild herbs. A good rule is that if you are not sure, do not use it.

Do not use essential oils in large doses as they are concentrated and may cause irritation in contact with the eyes or mucous membranes.

FORMS OF HERBAL PREPARATIONS

Tinctures:
: Made with the use of spirits where the herb cannot be heated or when the drug only gives up its principles to spirit.

Liquid extracts:
: Are the most concentrated form of the drug. They are made by concentrating the chemicals in liquid by evaporation, high pressure. 28gm of drug = 28gm of liquid

Infusions:
: Are made by pouring boiling water over the herb and letting it stand for half an hour and then straining the liquid off.

Decoctions:
: A decoction of the drug requires heat. Cold water is poured over the herb and then the mixture is boiled for twenty minutes, cooled and strained.

Percolation:
: A very effective way of obtaining the fluid, soluble part of a drug. This is obtained by allowing the fluid to drip through the drug time and time again in a percolator, until nearly all the soluble matter is extracted from the drug.

ALFALFA
Medicago sativa
Alfalfa is rich in Vitamins A, B2, B6, C, D and K. It picks up trace elements from the soil and contains eight essential amino acids and eight essential digestive enzymes. Alfalfa affects the stomach, liver and intestines and is an alternative nutritive tonic and antipyretic.

The flowers, leaves, and seeds are used. The alfalfa leaves can be steamed as vegetables or eaten in salads or soups. An infusion can also be made by using two teaspoons of dried alfalfa per cup of water. The seeds can be sprouted and used in a salad or on sandwiches.

Alfalfa is a hormone herb which, along with natural iodine, affects the parathyroids. These are small superficial glands situated on the back of the thyroid gland. These glands secrete the hormones calcitonin and parathoromone. These hormones act on the stabilisation of calcium in serum blood levels. Alfalfa also contains fat splitting enzymes and can be used in weight control. According to the ancient Chinese, excessive use will cause one to be thin. If between 10% to 20% of alfalfa is added to the formula of herbal combinations it increases the nutritive qualities of the formula.

ALOE
Aloe vera
The juice of this succulent can give quick relief to bites, burns, cuts, bruises. Taken internally it can be used for gastro-intestinal complaints such as colitis and ulcers.

ANISEED
Pimpinella anisum
The seed and leaf can be made into tea or used in cooking. It can be used as a weak diuretic, a laxative, relieving flatulence, an expectorant in treatment of bronchitis and asthma, and in aiding digestion.

BARBERRY
Berberis vulgaris
Commonly used to treat liver conditions, jaundice, and problems with the gall bladder. It can be used to treat nausea

and a mouthwash is effective for sore throats and lowering blood pressure.

BAYBERRY
Myrica cerifera
Commonly used to treat diarrhoea and mucous colitis. Bayberry is also as a gargle for sore throats and colds.

BEARBERRY (see Uva ursi)

BETONY
Betonica officinalis
It is useful in treating diarrhoea, it has mild sedative properties and can aid in the relief of headaches and anxiety, it has also been used in treatment of rheumatism and varicose veins. Beware of using the root as it may cause vomiting.

BLACK COHOSH
Cimicifuga racemosa
This herb can be used in the acute stage of rheumatoid arthritis and sciatica, it also relieves menstrual cramps. It is an effective stimulant for the heart and lowers high blood pressure but can also be used in cases of hysteria.

BETHROOT
Trillium erectum
It is used to treat menstrual problems and as a poultice it can be applied to ulcers and sores.

BLUEBERRY (BILBERRY)
Vaccinium myrtillus
The berries of this nutritious fruit can be dried and used for circulatory problems, the treatment of diabetes, burns, ulcers, inflamed gums, and catarrh. It also helps imporve night vision and is an antioxidant.

BOLDO
Peumus boldus
Stimulates the liver, the gall bladder, the digestive acids,

the pancreas, acts as a diuretic. It has been used in the treatment of urinary tract infections, and it has sedative properties.

BUCKTHORN BARK
Rhamnus cathartica
The bark of this plant can be used as a powerful diuretic and purgative which is used in cases of chronic constipation. Do not use the fresh bark as it is too strong.

CAMPHOR
Cinnamomum camphora
It is commonly used on inflammed joints but is also used in small doses as a sedative and for the reduction of fevers. It can be used as an antispasmodic for epilepsy. Applied externally it relieves sprains and strains. As an insect repellent it is useful.

CASCARA SAGRADA
Rhamnus purshiana
Cascara Sagrada affects the liver, gallbladder, colon, stomach and pancreas. It is a laxative, antispasmodic and hepatic tonic which is one of the safest tonic laxatives that can be used. It can be used in either the tincture or dried herb form.

Cascara increases liver, pancreas and bowel secretions and used in small, frequent dosages, restores the tone of the bowel and has a lasting, permanent effect. If a gentle laxative is required, use 20 drops of the tincture three times daily. If a more drastic action is required then the dose should be half a teaspoon full of the tincture three times daily.

Cascara is very valuable whenever haemorrhoids are associated with constipation and poor bowel function. It is also very useful for bowel related problems in combination with bayberry bark, rhubarb root, golden seal and raspberry leaves as a lower bowel tonic.

CASSIA
Cassia senna
Strong cathartic used for the treatment of constipation, the leaf is stronger than the fruit in usefulness.

CAYENNE
Capsicum annuum
As a dried, ground powder it can be used to improve circulation, digestion, help flatulence, and is sometimes used in the case of neuralgia and rheumatism. A weak solution can be used for a throat gargle. Mixed with slippery elm and used externally for chilblanes.

CELERY
Apium graveolens
The vegetable is recommended as a diuretic and appetite suppressant. The seeds are used for treating rheumatism and anxiety. Take Celery Complex.

CHICKWEED
Stellaria media
Rich in nutrients and vitamins A, B, and C, it eases constipation and inflammation of the digestive system. Externally it can be applied to haemorrhoids, skin irritations, eczema, bruises, rheumatic joints, and chilblains.

CLOVES
Eugenia caryophyllata
Its most well-known use is for toothache, and it is also used for flatulence and colic. Apply Oil of Cloves with a cotton bud to the ailing tooth.

COMFREY
Symphytum officinale
The foliage and root of this plant contain a nitrogenous, crystalline substance called allantoin which is a cell proliferant. Comfrey is a demulcent, alternative, expectorant, astringent and nutritive tonic. It has a soothing and healing effect upon every organ it comes in contact with. Comfrey is used externally for broken bones, sores and because of the above cell proliferant action, speeds up the healing of wounds. A poultice of freshly bruised leaves applied to a burn or wound, will increase the healing process and minimise inflammation. Since ancient times, Comfrey has also been known as the 'miracle herb', because not only is it a self proliferant, it also stops haemorrhages, is soothing to

inflamed tissues. NOTE: Comfrey is poionous and when taken in large amounts, or for long periods of time , it can accumulate. Seek advice from your naturopath.

CORN SILK
Zea mays
Combined with agrimony and made into a tea it is used to treat bed-wetting; alone it treats cystitis.

COUCH GRASS
Agropyron repens
Possessing antibiotic qualities, it acts as an antiseptic diuretic.

CRANESBILL (AMERICAN)
Geranium maculatum
Useful in cases of diarrhoea, haemorrhoids, peptic ulcers, and haemorrhaging in the digestive tract. It can be used as a mouthwash for mouth ulcers and sore throats. It is also used in treatment of thrush.

DANDELION
Taraxum officinale
Dandelion affects the kidneys, gallbladder, liver, pancreas and blood and contains the actives taraxcin, the monohydric alcohols taraxasterol and homotaraxasterol, fatty acid, sugar and insulin.
Dandelion would be one of the most prescribed herbs today, and its main use would be for liver complaints or as a diuretic. Dandelion stimulates the liver increasing its detoxifying action. Because of this action Dandelion is a valuable blood purifying herb and may be used in some skin diseases. Dandelion is also a very useful diuretic being much safer than juniper berry as it is non-irritant to the kidneys. The dandelion leaves can be eaten as part of a salad and will help prevent liver problems and gallstones. The dried roots are used to make a coffee substitute.

DEVIL'S CLAW
Harpagophytum procumbens
Devil's Claw in used to treat inflammation of joints, as in

arthritis, and also for mild analgesic properties. It is used to treat tennis elbow and when anti-inflammatory medicine is needed.

DILL
Anethum graveolens
Used fresh as a flavouring with potatoes, eggs, chicken, and fish, the seeds can be made into a tea to ease indigestion and in particular babies' colic.

DONG QUAI
Angelica sinensis
Dong quai can be used in the treatment of most female gynaecological ailments, in particular menstrual cramps, irregularity, a delayed flow during menstrual period. It also can be successfully used to treat hot flushes that often accompany menopause. It is nourishing to the blood, being rich in vitamin E and vitamin B12 and is also useful in the treatment of anaemia as well as being a valuable blood purifier.

Dong quai is also very useful in combination with other herbs such as black cohosh, queen of the meadow, red raspberry and bless thistle. I have found this combination excellent in the treatment of hormone imbalance and menopause problems.

ECHINACEA
Echinacea augustiflolia
This herb is used both internally and externally, for boils, acne, abscesses, severe bites, septicaemia, fevers, and in some cases it has been used to treat cancer. A dilator of peripheral blood vessels, it can also be used in prevention of viruses.

ELDER FLOWER
Sambuccus nigra
The flowers of the black elder are used as an ingredient in eye lotion and for skin complaints. They are mainly used to treat colds, sinus, chronic nasal catarrh with deafness, throat infections, and in combination with other herbs, it is used to treat constipation, diarrhoea, bronchitis, cystitis, and fluid retention.

EPHEDRA
Ephedra sinica
Used in bronchial asthma, hayfever, skin complaints, purifying the blood, urticaria. It contains the alkaloid ephedrine.

EUCALYPTUS
Eucalyptus globulus
The Tasmanian blue gum's oil is used externally for burns, cuts, ulcers, and sores. Inhaled, it clears the nose and lungs, aids bronchitis and asthma, and as a lozenge it relieves sore throats. It has a strong aroma, and acts as an antiseptic and disinfectant.

EUPHORBIA
Euphorbia hirta
Relaxes the bronchi and is used to treat asthma. The latex is used to treat warts.

EVENING PRIMROSE OIL
Oenothera biennis
The oil extracted from the leaves of this tree is used internally for coughs, colds, gastrointestinal and menstrual problems, as a sedative and for depression. The oil is used externally for skin eruptions and sores. Primrose oil can also help lower cholesterol and blood pressure.

EYEBRIGHT
Euphrasia officinalis
Used in eye lotion for conjunctivitis, it possesses anti-inflammatory qualities.

FENNEL
Foeniculum vulgare
A tea made from the seeds relieves flatulence, stimulates the pancreas, improving metabolism of fats and sugars. It is recommended for weight loss, nursing mothers, and diabetes and it is rich in minerals.

FENUGREEK
Trigonella foenum-graecum
Aids in bronchitis, catarrh, sinus, digestion of fatty foods and acne. A paste can be used for boils and wounds.

FEVERFEW
Tanacetum parthenium
Promotes menstruation, prevents migraine, headache, fever, tension.

GARLIC
Allium sativum
Well-known for its antibiotic qualities, garlic protects against the common cold, infectious diseases such as typhoid and dysentery, increases flow of bile from liver, can be used to treat tuberculosis, bronchitis and other respiratory disorders as well as treat intestinal ailments. It is also used in treatment of high blood pressure and hardening of the arteries. Garlic also lowers cholesterol.

GENTIAN
Gentian lutea
The root of the plant has been used to treat appetite and digestion, in such cases as debility and anorexia.

GINGER
Zingiber officinale
Treats nausea, motion sickness, colic and menstruation pain. It increases circulation and can cleanse the body by stimulating perspiration.

GINSENG
Panax ginseng
Gingseng is used to increase mental and physical efficiency and can reduce blood pressure and cholesterol and suppress development of cancer cells, bolstering the immune system, which also aids in the treatment of hepatitis B. Its action on the endocrine glands should increase vitamin and mineral utilisation. It has also been used to treat masculine sexual potency.

GLOBE ARTICHOKE
Cynara scolymus
Usually eaten as a delicacy, this vegetable treats jaundice and liver insufficiency and is a prophylactic against arteriosclerosis. Helps lower cholesterol.

GOLDEN SEAL
Hydrastis canadensis
Golden seal is taken internally for ulcers, dyspepsia, anorexia, gastritis, menstrual disorders. It causes oversecretion of mucous membranes, especially the uterus and relieves sinusitis. It is a tonic alternative, stimulant, antihaemorrhagic and laxative as well as being a powerful antiseptic and antibiotic which can be used for many diseases of the gastro-intestinal tract.

In combination with other herbs, golden seal stands on its own. A common example of this is the combination of golden seal and eyebright herb as an eye tonic. The herb bayberry may also be included in this formula. This formula is excellent when used to treat conjunctivitis and allergy eye problems.

As an eye-wash: 400 mg of the above dried herb combination to 1 cup of heated distilled water. Let stand for 1 hour, strain. It can now be used to bathe the eyes.

GRINDELIA
Grindelia robusta
Works as an expectorant and mild sedative for relief of respiratory tract infections and asthma.

GUAIACUM
Guaiacum officinale
Used to relieve the pain of rheumatism and arthritis, it works as an antiseptic and diuretic.

HAWTHORN
Crataegus oxyacanthoides
It is specifically used to treat the muscular action of the heart in conditions such as irregular heartbeat, palpitations, angina, arteriosclerosis, circulatory disorders, and blood pressure.

HOPS
Humulus lupulus
Used as a soporific to treat insomnia, anxiety, indigestion, and also for the relief of menstrual pain and neuralgia.

HOREHOUND
Marrubium vulgare
Beneficial for disorders of the gall bladder and the stomach, it can also be used to treat menstrual pain. It is specifically of use in bronchial disorders.

HORSERADISH
Cochlearia armoracia
Eaten raw, it stimulates digestion and treats bronchial disorders. It clears the head and relieves congestion and sinusitis and the related pain.

HORSETAIL
Equisitum arvense
Having a high silica content, horsetail can be used to clean pewter. A potent diuretic, it can be drunk as a tea to remove gall or kidney stones. It promotes coagulation and corpuscle growth, reducing internal and external bleeding.

IRISH MOSS
Chondrus crispus
Known as carrageen, Irish moss is a gelatin derived from seaweed and is used in pharmaceutical products. Its soothing properties are useful for bronchial and digestive irritations, and it is also nutritious and used for treating convalescents.

JUNIPER
Juniperus communis
Used internally as a urinary antiseptic and to stimulate appetite. The oil can be used in a vaporiser for bronchial infections. It is a diuretic which stimulates the kidneys.

KELP
Fucus vesiculosus
Kelp is used in the treatment of disorders of the thyroid gland and to treat overweight people; it contains iodine.

KOLA
Cola nitida
Kola is a heart stimulant and is high in caffeine. It is used to treat headaches, migraine and depression.

LIME FLOWERS
Tillia cordata
In combination with hawthorn and mistletoe, the flower can be used to treat hypertension, cardiac disease and high blood pressure.

LIQUORICE
Glycyrrhiza glabra
Liquorice root can be used as an expectorant in respiratory complaints, and it is well-known for its laxative properties. It is also used as an anti-inflammatory drug, possessing similar qualities to prednizone.

MILK THISTLE
Silybum marianum
Used as an appetite stimulant and an aid to digestion, the powdered seeds can be used in certain cardiovascular disorders. This herb has also been used to treat leg ulcers and varicose veins. It protects the liver from toxins and is used to treat hepatitis.

MULLEIN
Verbascum thapsus
Specifically used for respiratory disorders, working as an expectorant and a sedative. Externally an oil from the flowers can treat haemorrhoids, bruises, nappy rash and warts.

OATS
Avena sativa
Oats are nutritious and soothe the intestinal tract. The seeds are good for the heart and relieve nervous anxiety. The oatmeal is used for skin disorders and the dried straw is used as tea for chest complaints.

OLIVE OIL
Olea europaea
Apart from its culinary delights it has laxative properties, relieves ulcers, and it is believed to reduce cholesterol. Externally the oil is used on bruises, burns and bites, and softens dry skin and hair. Eating this flavoursome oil can enrich dry skin, relieve itchy scalp, add lustre to the hair.

PASSION FLOWER
Passiflora incarnata
Used in the treatment of insomnia, nervousness and anxiety, it is also employed to treat types of convulsion and also epilepsy. It is a sedative and a hypnotic. As an antispasmodic it is effective in the treatment of spasmodic asthma. Specifically it is most effective in treatment of insomnia and works well in combination with *Valeriana* and *Humulus*.

PEPPERMINT
Mentha x piperita
Gastro intestinal disorders are relieved by a cup of peppermint tea which stimulates internal circulation. It also relieves agitation and headaches. One of the most successful uses of peppermint tea is for the treatment of morning sickness. It is a great aid for flatulence. It is an internal antiseptic for the digestive system.

PLEURISY ROOT
Asclepias tuberosa
Specifically for the use of respiratory tract ailments such as pleurisy. It reduces pain and eases breathing. It is also used tin the treatement of bronchitis, pneumonia, and influenza. It can be combined with *Capsicum, Grindelia,* and *Lobelia* to treat cases of congestion of the lungs.

PSYLLIUM
Plantago psyllium
The mucilage on the seed swells when ingested and is effective for constipation, and also diarrohea. It helps lower blood cholesterol. Its most effective use is for Irritable

Bowel syndrome and in cases of colitis. It is sometimes used
to treat cystitis.

RASPBERRY
Rubus idaeus
The leaves in tea are beneficial for all womb-related
problems from menstruation to childbirth and can be drunk
daily. It cures diarrhoea. It can be used as a mouthwash in
cases of tonsilitis and with conjunctivitis it can be used as
an eye lotion.

RHUBARB
Rheum palmatum
The astringent root in small doses stops diarrhoea while in
large doses it works as a laxative.

ST JOHN'S WORT
Hypericum perforatum
Used for healing strains, sprains, ulcers, rheumatism,
haemorrhoids and ageing spots. Internally it is used for
respiratory and digestive disorders and, recently, in treatment
of AIDS patients.

SARSPARILLA
Smilax ornata
Useful to eliminate urea and uric acid from the blood, which
is necessary in the case of gout and rheumatism sufferers,
and occasionally psoriasis patients. It helps to improve the
health of the skin.

SCULLCAP
Scutellaria laterifolia
Specifically for spasms, excitability and epilepsy, it is also
used in combination with other herbs to treat insomnia,
headache, tension, and anxiety.

SENEGA
Polygala senega
Most commonly used as an expectorant to relieve bronchitis.

It also combines well with *Euphorbia* and with *Grindelia* in the treatment asthma and bronchitis.

SERENOA
Serenoa repens
Serenoa berries stimulate the lungs and genito-urinary systems and are used in recovering cases of chronic cystitis, bronchitis, catarrh, and sexual debility. It is used for the treatment of prostatic enlargement. As an endocrine agent and and anabolic agent it is used to treat cystitis and catarrh of the genito-urinary tract. It is also used in the treatment of sex hormone disorders.

SLIPPERY ELM
Ulmus fulva
Slippery Elm is a demulcent, emollient, antitussive and nutritive tonic. It affects the whole body, is rich in mucilage, acting rapidly by soothing the inflamed surfaces of a variety of mucous membranes and is especially beneficial for the lungs, stomach.and intestines. It is used to heal gastric ulcers.

Slippery Elm, because of its soothing qualities, can be used to help control diarrhoea as it quickly normalises bowel functions. It can be taken by either spreading the powdered bark over cereal or making it into gruel with water and a little honey. There are however, many commercially available slippery elm tablets and capsules which can be very convenient, depending on the condition to be treated and the age of the patient.

SPEARMINT
Mentha spicata
From the same genus as peppermint, spearmint aids digestion, but is not as strong and is suitable for colic in babies and children. It has diuretic properties.

TEA TREE OIL
Melaleuca alternifolia
An antiseptic white oil can be used to treat almost any skin disorder and used externally for ulcers, sores, wounds,

carbuncles, abscesses, fungi, including tinea, and as a gargle for throat infections.

THUJA
Thuja occidentalis
Used for relief of muscular aches and pains, it promotes menstruation, relieves headache, heart pain, and reduces swelling. It is used externally to treat warts.

Thuja is nerve stimulant which stimulates the heart and the uterus. It is particularly useful in cases of bronchitis with cardiac weakness. In treating uterine carcinomas and amenorrheoa is has been successful and it has been reported to be of value as an anti-carcinomatous agent. It can be used in combination with grindelia, senega, or lobelia for heart disease. Pregnant women should avoid thuja as it may cause contractions.

THYME
Thymus vulgaris
An antiseptic useful in urinary tract and digestive tract complaints. It stimuates the appetite, relieves flatulence and colic and is used specifically for the treatment of bronchitis and asthma. It may also be used to treat bronchitis, asthma, diarrhoea in children, and chronic gastritis.

UVA URSI (BEARBERRY)
Arctostaphylos uva-ursi
Specifically used in bladder and kidney infections and urinary tract disorders, success has been had in treatment of bronchitis, asthma, and urinary incontinence. Its main success as a urinary antiseptic is in the treatment of acute cystitis when highly acid urine is present.

VALERIAN
Valeriana officinalis
Valerian is well-known for its uses as a nervine and antispasmodic. Valerian can be used, in combination with a number of herbs, for many varying symptoms such as sleeplessness, nervousness, restlessness, irritability and anxiety states. One particular combination that I have used

in my clinic with great success is equal part of the fluid extracts of the herbs passion flower and valerian mixed with a small percentage of peppermint leaves.

WHITE WILLOW BARK
Salix alba
Salicin comes from the bark of this tree, and was the original aspirin, before it was produced synthetically. Salicin reduces inflammation and the pain of rheumatism, is good for oral inflammations, sores and wounds. Specifically it is used to treat rheumatoid arthritis and other systemic connective-tissue disorders which are inflamed. It may be combined with *Cimifuga, Apium* and *Guaiacum* in cases of rheumatoid arthritis. It also has fever reducing properties.

WINTERGREEN
Gaultheria procumbens
Readily absorbed through the skin, the oil treats aches and pains, including rheumatism and headaches. Its anti-inflammatory action makes it specifically useful in cases of rheumatoid arthritis. It is also used to treat sciatica and neuralgia.

FIRST AID HERBS

BULL ANT BITE: Take the root of the common bracken fern, break it in half and rub juice on the bite.

CHILBLAINS: Make a poultice using 3 parts slippery elm and 2 parts cayenne pepper. Apply to area.

CONJUNCTIVITIS: Make an infusion of eyebright and golden seal. Cool and filter. Use as eye wash morning and night.

CONSTIPATION: Take two tablets of Peritone with a large glass of water at bedtime.

HEADACHE: Take rosemary tea or 15 to 30 drops of the tincture as needed. Also white willow bark and betony.

HICCUPS: Take 10 mls of raspberry syrup (cordial) undiluted. Hiccups will stop instantly.

HIVES: Yarrow 28 ml, stinging nettles 28 ml, dandelion root 56 ml, golden seal 7 ml. Cover and simmer for 20 minutes in 1 litre of water. Dosage: take 1 tablespoon every 4 hours.

INDUCED VOMITING: Take Epacac as directed.

INFECTED WOUNDS: Apply a salve of golden seal and vitamin A ointment.

INSECT REPELLENT: Apply tea tree oil to all exposed areas. Avoid contact with eyes or mouth.

KIDNEY TONIC: Use 1:1 fluid extract. Corn silk 14 mls, parsley 14 mls, dandelion 14 mls, uva ursi 14 mls. Mix herbs and add 28 mls to 600 mls of distilled water and simmer for 20 minutes. Dosage: Take half to 1 cup of tea three times daily after meals as a general kidney and bladder tonic or as a diuretic to help dissolve kidney stones.

MIGRAINE
HEADACHES:

Formula 1: Dried herbs: fenugreek 1 part, thyme 1 part, feverfew 2 parts. Dosage: mix the dried herbs in equal parts and into '00' capsules, taking 2 capsules three times daily with meals to help prevent migraine headaches.

MENSTRUAL
CRAMPS:

Dried herbs: peony root 25%, liquorice 25%, dong quai 25%, red raspberry 25%. Mix herbs and using '00' gelatin caps, fill. Dosage: take 2 capsules 3 times daily with meals.

MORNING
SICKNESS:

Both red raspberry and peppermint tea can help here. Drink a cup of tea in the morning before getting out of bed and red raspberry tea at mealtimes for the rest of the day. Also take ginger and vitamin B6, 25 mg daily. Use the raspberry taa from the second trimester only.

STOMACH
AILMENTS:

Peppermint tea can help keep the digestion on an even keel and help prevent colic and flatulence.

SUNBURN:

Apply Aloe vera gel to the painful area when required. Cold tea and tomato can also relieve the pain.

TOOTHACHE:

Apply oil of cloves to the tooth cavity using a cotton bud.

ULCERS:

I have used this combination of herbs in my clinic for the treatment of stomach disorders and ulcers, with very successful results. Mix equal parts of the following dried herbs: slippery elm bark 33%, marshmallow root 33%, liquorice 33%. Dosage: Take 2 capsules just before meals 3 times daily. It must be stressed that a well-balanced diet, low in red meat and spices, with a larger portion of the diet being vegetables and whole grains should be eaten.

VAGINAL DOUCHE:

Slippery elm 28 gms, golden seal 28 gms, comfrey 28 gms, squawvine 28 gms, chaparral 28 gms. Take 30 gms of the herb mixture to 600 mls of water. Cover and simmer for half an hour, cool and strain. Add 14 mls of vinegar and use as douche once daily for 1 to 3 days.

VAGINITIS:

Using the dried herb mix together: golden seal 25%, squawvine 25%, chaparral 25%, Echinacea 25%. Fill '00' gelatin capsules with the herbal mix. Dosage: Take 2 capsules 3 times daily before meals.

PART IV
VITAMINS—MINERALS
AND THEIR USES

ALL ABOUT VITAMINS

Function In body	Signs of Possible Deficiency	Natural Food Sources
Vitamin A		
Antioxidant; shortens duration of disease (colds) and bursitis (inflammation) between bones and muscles; for treatment of acne and other skin eruptions; improves eyesight (prevents night blindness); healthy skin, hair, teeth and gums, mucus membranes.	Sinusitis and sore throat, colds, lung infection; night blindness, granules on eyelid.	cod liver oils, green and yellow vegetables, egg yolk, butter, cream

Function In body	Signs of Possible Deficiency	Natural Food Sources

B1 (Thiamine)

Helps in heart function; energy; calm nerves; promotes growth and aids carbohydrate metabolism; helps prevent travel sickness.

Anorexia; lack of energy; cardiovascular disorders; mental confusion; peripheral paralysis; grooves in tongue; depression; low blood pressure; lack of energy; cardiovascular disorders; poor memory;

peanuts, soybeans, meats, brewer's yeast (available in flakes or tablets), molasses, bran

B (Riboflavin)

Aids in growth and reproduction; helps eliminate sore and cracked mouth, lips and tongue; necessary for healthy skin, nails, hair; promotes body's use of oxygen; helps alleviate eye fatigue.

Lesions on lips, mouth, skin; cataracts; eyes sensitive to light; burning eyes, scaling around nose.

milk, fish, eggs, kidney, liver, brewer's yeast

B3 (Niacin Nicotinic Acid)

Aids in digestion; helps relieve headaches; necessary for healthy nervous system; increased circulation; essential for synthesis of sex hormones, cortisone, thyroxine, and insulin; helps reduce cholesterol.

Negative personality changes; nervousness; bad breath; high cholesterol; arteriosclerosis.

dates, figs, prunes, wheat, wheat germ, avocadoes, fish, eggs, whole wheat, lean meats, brewer's yeast dessicated liver

Function In body	Signs of Possible Deficiency	Natural Food Sources
B5 (Pantothenic Acid) Helps synthesis of cholesterol; necessary for growth and reproduction; skin and hair health; relieves stress; aids nervous system; prevents premature ageing.	Muscle cramps; anemia; severe eczema; dry skin and wrinkles; hypoglycaemia; burning feet.	molasses, grains, nuts, liver, egg yolk, green vegetables, whole grains, wheat germ, brewer's yeast, organ meats
B6 (Pyridoxine) Absorption of vitamin B12; reduces muscle spasms; necessary for production of red blood cells; works as a diuretic; essential for production of hydrochloric acid and utilisation of magnesium.	Convulsions; anemia; muscular weakness; loss of hair; fluid retention.	brewer's yeast, liver, eggs, blackstrap molasses, cantaloupe, cabbage, germ, beef, wheat bran, all meats
Folic acid (Folacin) Aids in protein metabolism; essential for formation of red blood cells; is a coenzyme needed for formation of nucleic acid.	Impaired growth and cell division; anaemia; greying hair; inflammation of the tongue.	pumpkins, beans, whole wheat, egg yolk, carrots, liver, deep green leafy vegetables, cantaloupe, apricots, dark rye flour, brewer's yeast.

Function In body	*Signs of Possible Deficiency*	*Natural Food Sources*
B12 (Cabalamin)		
Aid folic acid in the synthesis of choline; regenerates red blood cells; utilises fats, carbohydrates and proteins; increases energy; promotes growth and appetite; helps iron function.	Severe deficiency causes anaemia, brain damage, poor memory; weakness in legs and arms.	milk, cheese, eggs, liver, kidney, muscle meats.
B13 (Orotic acid)		
Metabolises folic acid and vitamin B12; aids in treatment of multiple sclerosis; could prevent liver problems and premature ageing.	Liver disorders; premature ageing.	root vegetables, whey
B15 (Pangamic acid)		
Relieves symptoms of angina; protects against pollutants; aids in protein synthesis; lowers cholesterol levels; extends cell life span; aids in circulation.	Heart disease; oxygenation of living cells; glandular and nervous disorders.	pumpkin seeds, brewer's yeast, sesame seeds, whole brown rice, whole grains
B17 (Laetrile)		
Forms healthy cells.	May lead to diminishing resistance to cancer.	nectarines, plums, apricots, apples, cherries

Function In body	Signs of Possible Deficiency	Natural Food Sources
Biotin		
Essential for metabolism of fats, carbohydrates and proteins; eases muscle pain; necessary for healthy skin; aids in keeping hair colour and preventing baldness.	Anorexia; dry, scaly skin; depression; nausea; muscular pain; lack of energy.	nuts, fruits, milk, kidney, beef liver, egg yolk, brewer's yeast
Choline		
Helps control cholesterol level; aids memory; necessary for function of kidneys and liver; assists nerve impulses; helps for lecithin; helps prevent gallstones.	Fatty degeneration of the liver; hardening of arteries; stomach ulcers (bleeding).	liver, organ meats, green leafy vegetables; brewer's yeast, egg yolks, soybeans, lecithin.
Inositol		
Helps lower cholesterol level; nourishment of brain cells; promotes healthy hair; helps body produce lecithin cells; promotes healthy hair.	High cholesterol; unhealthy brain cells; eczema; constipation; hair loss.	grapefruit, cabbage, blackstrap molasses, beans, wheat germ, liver, peanuts, lima, cantaloupe, raisins, beef, brains and heart, lecithin, brewer's yeast

	Signs of	
Function	*Possible*	*Natural*
In body	*Deficiency*	*Food Sources*

PABA (Para Aminobenzoic Acid)

| Helps form blood cells; keeps skin healthy and young; helps form folic acid; sun screening properties; utilises protein; stimulates intestinal bacteria. | Eczema; thinning hair; grey hair. | molasses, rice, bran, whole grains, liver, kidney, brown rice, wheat germ |

C (Ascorbic Acid)

| Antioxidant; holds body cells together; aids prevention of infection; helps decrease blood cholesterol; aids healing process; reduces allergies; reduces common cold symptoms; vital for formation of bones and collagen. | Scurvy; bruise easily; allergies; inflammation and infections; stress. | sprouting seeds, tomatoes, green peppers, rose hips, fresh citrus, fruits, acerola berries, vegetables. |

D

| Helps prevent colds; aids in assimilating vitamin A; utilises calcium and phosphorus. | Deformity of bones; rickets; tooth decay. | tuna, whole milk and dairy products, cod liver oil, sardines |

Function In body	Signs of Possible Deficiency	Natural Food Sources
Vitamin E (Tocopherol)		
Keeps fats from becoming rancid when exposed to air; fertility and normal production; aids in utilisation of vitamin A; helps prevent heart and blood diseases; antioxidant.	Reproductive disorders; anaemia; muscle degeneration and destruction of red blood cells; premature ageing; heart disease; cancer.	whole grains, wheat germ oil, cold-pressed vegetable oils.
Vitamin F		
Gives some protection against harmful x-rays; aids in weight loss; unsaturated fats (liquid oils) help burn saturated fats (solids); helps regulate blood clotting.	Acne; eczema; brittle hair; varicose veins.	sunflower seeds, unsaturated fats (vegetable oils), wheat germ, cod liver oil
Vitamin K (Menadione)		
Promotes proper blood clotting; helps prevent internal bleeding; helps liver function.	Sprue; sore, red tongue, anaemia; celiac disease; nose bleeds.	soybean oil, kelp, leafy green vegetables, yoghurt, alfalfa, soybean oil, egg yolk, cod liver oil, molasses
Vitamin P (Flavonoids)		
Increases capillary strength; works with vitamin C.	Causes infections and bruises.	rose hips, yellow substance of citrus fruits, lemons, buckwheat, rose hips

Function In body	*Signs of Possible Deficiency*	*Natural Food Sources*
Vitamin T		
Helps blood coagulation and formation of platelets.	Anaemia and haemophilia can result.	sesame seeds, egg yolks.
Vitamin U		
Helps ulcers heal.	Ulcers may occur.	raw cabbage, sauerkraut

WHAT MINERALS DO

Function In body	Signs of Possible Deficiency	Natural Food Sources
Calcium		
There is more calcium in the body than any other mineral. Calcium and phosphorus work together. One is not effective without the other. Corrects allergic reactions; metabolizes iron; maintains strong bones and teeth; blood coagulation; regulates heart; alleviates insomnia; aids nervous system and muscles.	Osteoporosis; aching limbs; vascular disorders; extreme deficiency causes poor teeth; causes rickets (malformed bones), inflammation of and weak bones.	sesame seeds, figs, raisins, milk and powdered milk, blackstrap molasses, cheese, green vegetables, soybeans, yoghurt, dried beans, sardines and salmon (with bone), sunflower seeds, peanuts and walnuts
Chromium		
Helps prevent high blood pressure; helps prevent diabetes; aids growth.	Arteriosclerosis (hardening of the arteries); diabetes (disorder of either the pancreas or the hypothalamus glands).	brewer's yeast, meat, corn oil, shellfish, chicken, clams
Chloride		
Chlorinated water destroys intestinal bacteria. aids digestion; promotes healthy teeth and hair.	Poor digestion, poor teeth and hair.	yoghurt, salt, kelp, olives

Function In body	*Signs of Possible Deficiency*	*Natural Food Sources*
Cobalt		
Builds red blood cells; helps prevent anaemia		meat, milk, oysters, kidneys, clams, liver
Copper		
Can reach blood-stream 15 minutes after ingestion Essential for Vit. C utilisation Aids in pigmentation factor of hair and skin aids in effective iron absorption	Edema (excessive fluid in tissues; abnormal swelling) Anaemia	shrimp and most dried beans, peas, calf and beef liver, prunes, peas, whole wheat
Fluorine		
The tissue strengthener Synthetic fluorine is toxic poison, Natural fluorine is beneficial Strengthens teeth and bones	Tooth decay	egg white, seafood, radishes, gelatin, cabbage, whole wheat, lettuce, garlic, beets
Iodine		
Healthy hair, nails skin and teeth; helps burn excess fat; improves mental alacrity; promotes growth; gives energy.	Hair loss; lack of energy; hypothyroidism; excessive weight gain; goitre.	Irish moss, vegetables grown in rich soil, kelp, seafood, onions.

Function In body	Signs of Possible Deficiency	Natural Food Sources

Iron

The blood mineral Coffee and tea inhibits iron absorption; essential to body's energy producing functions; necessary for metabolisation of B vitamins; required for production of haemoglobin (red blood corpuscles); myoglobin (red pigment in muscles) and certain enzymes.

Occurs in blood disorders; inflammations; haemorrhages and anaemia.

kelp, brown rice, soybean, pork liver, parsley, beef kidney, heart and liver, apricots, red meat, molasses, egg yolks, raisins, oysters, oatmeal, nuts, beans, asparagus, beets

Manganese

Aids digestion; improves reflexes and memory; reduces irritability and eliminates fatigue.

Improves poor digestion and fatigue.

egg yolk, whole grains, beets, nuts, green leafy vegetables, peas

Magnesium

Called the nerve mineral it converts blood sugar into energy; aids calcium and vitamin C metabolism, as well as phosphorus, sodium and potassium; effective nerve and muscle function.

Aids relief of tics, spasms, headaches, muscle twitchings, poor teeth, kidney and gallstones, depression, and heart disease.

sesame seeds, whole wheat, apples, figs, dark green vegetables, lemons, seeds, grapefruit, corn nuts

Function In body	*Signs of Possible Deficiency*	*Natural Food Sources*
Phosphorus		
The mood mineral present in every cell; nervous system tonic; aids in metabolism of fats and starches; bone and tooth structure; heart regularity; transfer of nerve impulses; kidney function.	Relieves anxiety and osteoporosis; loss of strength; sensitivity; rickets; pyorrhea (disease of bones around teeth).	mung beans, lentils, brown rice, fish, nuts and seeds, poultry, eggs, whole grains, meat
Potassium		
The brain mineral, destroyed by alcohol, caffeine, sugar, diuretics, and over-cooking; aids in allergy treatment; aids in sending oxygen to brain; assists in reducing blood pressure; helps dispose of body wastes.	Indicated by irritability, noise sensitivity, yawning, hysteria, hypoglycaemia, and edema.	lettuce, dandelion, barley, citrus fruits, whole grains, watercress, potatoes, green leafy vegetables, bananas, mint leaves, sunflower seeds
Selenium		
Works with vitamin E; males need more than females; works as an antioxidant; alleviates hot flashes; slows down ageing; protects against certain cancers; prevents dandruff.	Premature ageing is a sign.	garlic, wheat germ, broccoli, bran, tomatoes, tuna, onions

Function In body	Signs of Possible Deficiency	Natural Food Sources
Sodium		
The fluid mineral regulates body water balance; aids in preventing heat prostration or sunstroke, and helps nerves and muscles function properly.	Heartburn, oyspepsia, possible neuralgia, and impaired carbo-hydrate digestion are all indications.	kelp, figs, coconut, salt, kidney, brains, carrots, bacon, beets, dried beef, arti-chokes, bacon, shell-fish
Sulphur		
The purifying min-eral helps prevent acne and skin dis-ease; promotes healthy hair, skin and nails; helps combat bacter-ial infection; maintains proper brain function and liver and bile secre-tion.	Effects are liver ail-ments, jaundice, yel-lowish skin and associated headache; skin disease, sores, psoriasis, boils, acne.	raspberries, cabbage, fish, beef, dried beans, eggs
Zinc		
Decrease in choles-terol deposits; forma-tion of body insulin; helps avoid prostate problems; maintains body's acid-alkaline balance; accelerates healing; tones repro-ductive organs; brain function.	Acne and skin disor-ders show deficiency; slow wound healing; enlarged prostate galnd; arteriosclerosis.	nonfat dry milk, red meat, eggs, wheat germ, pumpkin seeds, brewer's yeast

| *Signs of* |
| *Function*   *Possible* | *Natural* |
| *In body*   *Deficiency* | *Food Sources* |

Trace minerals   Alfalfa
aluminium, boron,
bromine, chromium,
molybdenum, nickel,
silicon, silver and
vanadium
All are necessary for
proper bodily
function

PART V
UNDERSTANDING
MEDICAL
TERMINOLOGY

Many people have asked me if I would explain some of the medical symbols and abbreviations used in Allopathic and Naturopathic medical writing.

It is interesting to see all the different terminologies used by the different modalities. To remember them all would be quite difficult. Homoeopathy, herbalism, naturopathy and allopathic medicine often use different terminology and symbols to define diseases and medication.

It is important to remember that although there may seem to be a difference in terminology all are accurate and correct. No one modality has the sole right to the only answer, after all, be it an anodyne, analgesic or pain reliever, the results are the same. Following is a list of common symbols used by ambulance officers, hospitals and pharmacists.

Δ DISEASE	# FRACTURE	♀	FEMALE
α ALPHA	β BETA	2/365	2 DAYS
† DEATH	i ONE	2/7	2 DAYS
ii TWO	♂ MALE	6/52	6 WEEKS
R.C. before meals	b.d. twice daily	q.d.s.	four times daily
P.C. after meals			
MANE morning		t.i.d.	three times daily
NOCTE night		t.d.s.	

DEFINITION OF TERMINOLOGY

Terminology is a study of words that are used to communicate ideas and facts. The origin of most medical words comes from

Latin and Greek languages, e.g. NEPHRO Greek = KIDNEY
                                   OSTEO   Greek = BONE
                                   CALCIUM Latin = CALCIUM

The suffixes and prefixes are also very important as they can give a more accurate description of the disease or condition.

Some examples of the use of suffixes are:

SUFFIX	EXAMPLE OF USE MEANING
ORRHAGIA—an excessive bursting forth	MEN/ORRHAGIA—monthly/excessive blood
CYTE—cell	LEUCO/CYTE—white cell
SCOPY—to view	GASTRO/SCOPY—stomach/to view
MALACIA—softening	OSTEO/MALACIA—bone/softening
EMESIS—vomiting	HYPER/EMESIS—excessive vomiting
PEPSIA—digestion	DYS/PEPSIA—bad/digestion
ALGIA—pain condition	NEUR/ALG/IA—nerve pain condition
PLASTY—surgical repair	ARTHRO/PLASTY—joint repair

Prefixes of words are also important as they can denote colour, position and numbers, etc.

Some examples of PREFIXES and their use follows:

PREFIX	MEANING	WORD EXAMPLE MEANING
A	without/lack of	A/PATHY—without/feeling
AMBI	both	AMBI/DEXTROUS—using both hands
BI	twice	BI/LATERAL—both sides
BRADY	slow	BRADY/CARDIA—slow heart (beat)
CONTRA	opposite/against	CONTRA/CEPTION—prevent conception
DYS	difficult/bad	DYS/PNEA—difficult breathing

Prefixes that denote colours:

                     AURUM—golden
                     LEUCO—white
                     ERYTHRO—red
                     POLIO—grey
                     CYANO—blue

MELAN—black
XANTH—yellow

As you can see, by combining prefixes, root word and suffixes, it is possible to form a word to describe a condition or disease. By bringing together a number of signs and symptoms and their terminology, we can actually construct a word or break it down to determine its meaning.

   i.e.   POLIO—grey—prefix
          MYEL—spinal cord—root
          ITIS—inflammation of—suffix

The constructed word now is Poliomyelitis which is an inflammatory disease affecting the grey matter of the spinal cord.

This is just a short look at Medical Terminology and I am sure that as you study it you will find that it is not as mysterious as it first appears.

A good idea would be to undertake a course in Medical Terminology. These are run by the Health Department usually in conjunction with a local hospital. Your *Taber's Cyclopedic Medical Dictionary* is also a good source of information on construction and dissemination of words used in medical terminology.

REFERENCES

ACNE
Ayres, S. Jnr, Mihan, R. 'Acne Vulgaris and Lipid Peroxidation: New Concepts in Pathogenesis and Treatment': *Int. J. Dermatol*, 17, p 305, 1978

Dowining, D.T., Stewart, M.E., Wetz, P.W., Strauss, J.S. 'Essential Fatty Acids and Acne' *J. Am. Acad. Dermatol* 14: pp 221-5, 1986

Hubler, W.R. 'Unsaturated Fatty Acids in Acne' *Arch. Dermatol* pp 644-6, 1959

Metal, A. 'Serum Zinc in Acne Vulgaris' *Int. J. Dermatol* 21, p 481, 1982

Mihanr, A. 'Acne Vulgaris: Therapy Directed at Pathophysiologic Defects ' *Cutis* 28, pp 41-2, 1981

ALCOHOL
DiLuzio, N.R. 'A mechanism of the acute ethanol-induced fatty liver and the modification of liver injury by antioxidants.' *Lab. Invest.* 15: pp 50-60, 1966

Guenther, R.M. 'Role of nutritional therapy in alcoholism treatment'. *Int. J. Biosocial Res.* 4 (1): pp 5-18, 1983

Majumdar, S.K, et al. 'Blood vitamin status (B1, B2, B6, folic acid and B12) in patients with alcoholic liver disease' *Int. J. Vitamin, Res.* 52 (3): pp. 266-71, 1982

Yunice, A.A., et al. 'Ethanol-ascorbate interrelationship in acute and chronic alcoholism in guinea pig' *Proc. Soc. Exp. Biol. Med.* 177: pp 262-71, 1984

ALLERGIES
Kaminura, M. 'Anti-inflammatory Activity of Vitamin E' *J. Vitamol* 18 (4), pp 204-9, 1972

Werbach, R. Nutritional Influences on Illness, A Sourcebook of Clinical Research (1988)

ANALGESICS
British Herbal Pharmacopoeia pp 111, 184 (British Herbal Medicine Association, West Yorkshire, 1983)

Budok 'Use of D-phenylalanine, An Enkephalinase Inhibitor, In the Treatment of Intractable Pain' *Adv. Pain Res. and Therapy* 5: pp 305-308, 1983

Martindale, The Extra Pharmocopoeia 29th edition, (Pharmaceutical Press, London, 1983)

ANTIOXIDANTS
Florence, T.M. 'Dietary need for antioxidants' *Clinically Speaking* 2: July 1990

Gey, K.F., Brubacher, et al ' Plasma levels of antioxidant vitamins in relation to heart disease and cancer' *Am. J. Clin. Nutr.* 45: pp 1363-77, 1987

Pauling, L. <u>How to Live Longer and Feel Better </u> (Avon Books, New York, 1986)

ARTHRITIS

<u>British Herbal Pharmacopoeia</u> , pp 28, 107, 111, 184, 193 (British Herbal Medicine Association, West Yorkshire, 1983)

Kremer, J.M. 'Effects of Manipulation of Dietary Fatty Acids on Clinical Manifestations of Rheumatoid Arthritis' *Lancet* 1: pp 184-7, 1985

Horrobin, D.F. 'The Importance of Gamma Linolenic Acid and Prostoglandic E in Human Nutrition and Medicine' *J. Holistic Med.* 3, pp 118-139, 1981

'Calcium Pantothenate in Arthritic Conditions. A Report from the General Practitioner Research Group' *Practioner* 224: pp 208-11, 1980

ASTHMA

<u>British Herbal Pharmacopoeia</u> pp 88, 104, 106, 212 (British Herbal Medicine Association, West Yorkshire, 1983)

Pizzorno and Murray 'A Textbook of Natural Medicine' *Asthma* II (vi) 1988

Horrobin, D.F. <u>Omega-6, Essential Fatty Acids, Pathophysiology and Roles in Clinical Medicine</u> (1990)

BITES AND STINGS

<u>Australian First Aid</u> St John Ambulance pp 180-199, 1, 1990

BRONCHITIS

Mills, S. <u>The Dictionary of Modern Herbalism</u> (Lothian, London, 1985)

CAFFEINE

'Coffee drinking and acute myocardial infarction.' *Lancet* 2: pp 1278-9, 1972

Dubey, P., et al. *Dig. Dis. & Su.* 29(3): pp 202-06, 1984

La Croix, A.Z., et al. 'Coffee Consumption and the incidence of coronary heart disease.' *New Engl. J. Med.* 315 (16): pp 977-82, 1986

CALCIUM

Ashmead 'Chelated Mineral' *Nut. P.S.*, 1981

Carafoli <u>Calcium and Cell Regulation</u> (Biochemical Society, London, 1974)

'Does Calcium Supplementation Prevent Post-Menopausal Bone Loss?' *The New England Journal of Medicine* 316 (4) : 22 Jan. 1987

Horsman, A., Gallagher, J.C., Simpson, M., Nordin, B.E.C.

'Prospective Trial of Oestrogen and Calcium in Postmenopausal Women' *Brit. Med. J.* 2: pp 789-792, 1977

New England Journal of Medicine 313: pp 70-73, 11 July 1985

Nordin, B.E.C., Peacock, M., Aaron, J. 'Osteoporosis and Osteomalacia' *Clin. Endocrinal Metab.* 9: 1980

'Toxicity of the Essential Minerals', Division of Nutrition, Bureau of Foods, Dept of Health, Education and Welfare, Washington

Zemel *J. Nut* 111 (2): pp 315-324, 1981

CANCER

Belmans 'Onion and garlic oil inhibit tumor growth.' *Carginogenesis* 4 (8): pp 1063-5, 1983

Carper, J. 'Fish oil and cancer', *The Courier Mail,* 6 June 1990

Clark, L.C. and Combs, 'Selenium compounds and the prevention of cancer. Research needs and public implications'. *J. Nutr.* 166: pp 170-176, 1986

Eosti (ed.), Florence, T.M., The role of Free Radicals in Cancer and Aging, in Trace Elements, Micronutrients and Free Radicals, (Humana Press, New York 1990)

Florence, T.M., 'Cancer and Ageing, The free radical connection,' *Chem. Australia,* 50: pp 166-174, 1983

Gey, K.F., Brubacher, G.B., and Stahelin, H.B., 'Plasma levels of antioxidant vitamins in relation to heart diseases and cancer. *Amer. J. Clin. Nutr,* 45: pp 1363-1377, 1987

Graham, S. et. al. 'Dietary factors in the epidemiology of cancer of the larynx'. *A.M.J. Epidemoil.* 113 (6): pp 675-80, 1981

Horrobin, D. 'Med. Hypotheses' 6: pp 469-86, 1980

Menkes, M.S., et. al. 'Serum Beta Carotene, Vitamins A and E, Selenium and the risk of Lung Cancer'. *New Engl. J. Med.* 315: p 1250, 1986

Modan, B. et. al. *J. National Cancer Instit,* 55: pp 15-18, 1975

'Nutrition, Diet and Cancer', The National Academy of Sciences, 1982

Stich, H.F., et. al. 'A pilot beta carotene intervention trial with invits using smokeless tobacco. *Int. J. Cancer* 36: p 321, 1985

CHILDREN'S VITAMINS

Lancet January, 1988

COLD HANDS AND FEET

Ayres Jnr., S. 'Raynaud's Phenomenon, Scleroderma and Calcinosis Cutis: Response to Vitamin E' *Cutis* 11, pp 54-62, 1973

British Herbal Pharmacopoeia pp 47-48, (British Herbal Medecine Association, West Yorkshire, 1983)

'International Symposium: Considerazioni Cliniche e Valutazioni Minerva Medica' 64 (supplement 79): pp 4060-201, 1973

COLD SORES
Fitzherbert, J 'Gential Herpes and Zinc' *Med. J. Aust.* 1: p 399, 1979
Griffith, R., Norins, A. 'A Multicentred Study of Lysine Therapy in Herpes Simplex Infection' *Dermatol* 156: pp 257-67, 1978
Terazhealmy, G., Bottomley, W. and Pellu, G. 'The Use of Water Soluble Bioflavonoid - Abscorbic Acid Complex in the Treatment of Recurrent Herpes Labialis' *Oral Surg.* 45: pp 56-62, 1978

CRAMPS
National Dietary Survey of Adults, Dept of Community Service and Health, Australia, pp 68, 76, 1987

CROHN'S DISEASE
Barrett, K.E., Tashof and Metcalf D.D. 'Inhibition of 1 gram emediated most cells degranulation by sulphasalazine' *J. Pharmacol.* 104: pp 279-81, 1985
British Herbal Pharmocopoeia pp 222-23, 1983
Lee, T.H., Hoover, R.L., Williams, J.D. et al 'Effect of dietary enrichment with eicosapentainoic and docosahexanoic acids on in vitro neutrophil and monocyte leukotriene generation and neutrophil function' *New Eng. J. Med.* 312: pp 1271-24, 1985
Llyod-Still, J. and Green, O.C. 'A clinical scoring system for chronic inflammatory bowel disease in children' *Dig. Dis. Science* 24: pp 620-24, 1979
Mayberry, J.F., Rhodes, J. and Newcombe, R.G. 'Increased sugar consumption in Crohn's Disease' *Digestion* 20: 323-6, 1980
Morain, Segal and Levi 'Elemental diet as a primary treatment of acute Crohn's Disease; a controlled trial' *B. R. Med. J.* 279: pp 764-76, 1979
Smith, M.A. et al 'Food intolerance, atopy, and irritable bowel syndrome' *Lancet* 2: p 1064, 9 Nov. 1985
Wakefield, A.J., Dhillon, A.P. et al 'Pathogenesis of Crohn's disease: multifocal gastointestinal infraction' *Lancet* pp 1057-62, Nov. 1989

DIABETES MELLITUS
Peifer, J.J., Holman, R.T. 'Essential Fatty Acid, Diabetes and Cholesterol' *Arch. Biochem. Bio. Phys* 57: pp 520-1, 1965
Potter, J., 'Glucose Metabolism in Glucose Tolerant Older People During Chromium Supplementation' *Metabolism* 34: pp 199-204, 1985
Som, S. 'Abscorbic Acid Metabolisms in Diabetes Mellitus' *Metabolism* 30 (6): pp 572-7, 1981
Tarui, S. 'Studies of Zinc Metabolism: Effect of the Diabetic

State on Zinc Metabolism: A Clinical Aspect' *Endocrin.* (Japan) 10: pp 9-15, 1963

DIVERTICULITIS

British Herbal Pharmocopoiea pp 222-3, 1983

Manning, A.P. 'Wheat Fibre and Irritable Bowel Syndrome: A Controlled Trial' *Lancet* 2: p 417, 1977

Niv, M. 'Yoghurt in the treatment of infantile diarrhoea' *Clin. Ped.* 2: pp 407-11, 1963

Rees, W.R.W. 'Treating Irritable Bowel Syndrome with Peppermint Oil' *Brit. Med. J.* 6 Oct. 1979

EPILEPSY

British Herbal Pharmocopoeia pp 193-4, 1983

Crayton, J.W. 'Epilepsy Precipitated by Food Sensitivity. Report of a Case with Double-Blind Placebo-controlled assessment' *Clin. Electroencephalo.* 2 (4): pp 192-8, 1981

Mantovani, J. 'Effects of taurine on seizures and growth hormone release in epileptic patients' *Arch. Neuro.* 35: p 672, 1979

Nakazawa. M/ 'High dose vitamin B6 therapy in infantile spasms. The effects and adverse reactions.' *Brain and Development* 5(2): p 193, 1983

Roach, E.S., Carlin, L. 'N-dimethylglycine for epilepsy' (letter to ed.) *N. Eng. Med. J.* 307: 1081-82, 1982

Shoji, Y, 'Serum magnesium and zinc in epileptic children' *Brain and Dev.* 5 (2): p 200, 1983

GALLSTONES

Breneman, J.C. 'Allergy elimination diet as the most effective gallbladder diet' *Ann. Allergy* 26: p 83, 1968

British Herbal Pharmacopoeia pp 206-8, 1983

Dam, H. *Acta Path. Microbiol. Scand.* 30: p 256, 1952

Faber, K. 'The Dandelion - Taraxum officinale' *Pharmazie* 13: pp 423-35, 1958

Jenkins, S. A. 'Vitamin C and gallstone formation, a preliminary report' *Experientia* 33: pp 1616-7, 1977

Mowrey, D.B. The Scientific Validation of Herbal Medicine (Cormorant Books, 1986)

HAWTHORN

Deutsche Medical Wchnschr 76: p 211, 1951

New England Journal of Medicine 14 Dec. 1967

Pharmazie p 141, 1951

HEADACHES

British Herbal Pharmocopoeia pp 39-40, 184-5, 1983

Greden, J.F. 'Caffeine Withdrawal Headache: A clinical profile' *Psychosomatics* 21: pp 411-18, 1980

Shirlow, M.J., Mathers, C.D. 'A study of caffeine consumption and symptom, indigestion, palpitation, tremor, headache and insomnia.' *Int. J. Epidemiol* 14(2): pp 239-48, 1985

HEART DISEASE
Bordia, A.K., Verma, S.K. 'Garlic found to regress atherosclerosis in rabbits' *Artery* 7: p 428, 1980
Burch, G.E., Giles, T.D. 'The importance of magnesium deficiency in cardiovascular disease' *Lancet* 1: pp 1044-6, 1977
Erst, E. 'Garlic and blood lipids' *British Med. J.* 291: p139, 1985
Herold, P.M. 'Fish Oil Consumption and Decreased Risk of Cardio-Vascular Disease; A Comparison of Findings from Animal and Human Feeding Trials' *Am. Nut. J.* 43: pp 566-98, 1986
Herman, W.J. 'The effect of tocopherol on high-density lipoprotein cholesterol: a clinical observation' *Am. J. Clin. Path.* 72: pp 848-52, 1979
Lady Cilento You don't have to live with ailing heart and blood vessels 1977

HYPOGLYCAEMIA
Anderson, R.A 'Chromium supplementation of humans with hypoglycaemaia' *Fed. Proc.* 43: p 471, 1984
Curry, D.L. 'Magnesium modulation of glucose induced insulin secretion by the perfused rat pancreas' *Endocrinology* 101: p 203, 1977
Sanders, L.R. 'Refined carbohydrate as a contributing factor in reactive hypoglycaemia' *Southern Med. J.* 75: p 1072, 1982

IMMUNE SYSTEM
Bland, J.S. Chronic Infections and Immune Function 1988
Cathcard, R.F. 'Vitamin C in the treatment of Acquired Immune Deficiency Syndrome (AIDS)' *Med. Hypotheses* 14: pp 423-33, 1984
Cavallito, C.J., Bailey, J.H. 'Allicin, the antibacterial principle of Allium sativum. Isolation, physical properties and antibacterial action.' *J. Am. Chem. Soc.* 66: p 1950-51, 1944
Elamin, I., Elnim, Syed, A., Abdel, G., Mossa, J. 'The antimicrobial activity of garlic and onion extracts' *Pharmazie* 38: p-747, 1983
Huddleson, I.F., Dufrain, J., Barrons, K.C., Geifel, M. 'Anti-bacterial substances in plants' *J. Am. Vet. Med. Assoc.* 105: pp 394-7, 1944
Keith, M.D., Pelletier, O. 'Abscorbic acid concentration in leukocytes and selected organs of guinea pigs in response to

the increasing abscorbic acid intake' *Am. J. Clin. Nut.* 27: p 368, 1974

Mose, J. 'Effect of Echinacin on Phagocytosis and Natural Killer Cells' *Med. Welt.* 34: pp 1423-33, 1984

Pizzorno and Murray John Bastyr Textbook of Natural Medicine: Echinacea *Echin.* V, 1, 1985

Takahashi,I., Nakanishi, S., 'Hypericin and pseudohypericin specifically inhibit protein kinose C; Possible relation to their antiretroviral activity' *Biochem. Biophysical Res, Comm.* 165 (3): pp 1207-12, 1989

Vahera, S.B., Rizwan, M., Khan, J.A. 'Medical Uses of Common Indian Vegetables' *Planta Med.* 23: pp 381-93, 1973

Wagner, V., Proksch, A., Riess-Maurer, I 'Immunostimulating Polysaccharides (heteroglycanes) of Higher Plants Preliminary Communications' *Arzneim Forsch* 34: pp 659-60, 1984

Tsai, Y., Cole, L.L., Davis, L.E., Lockwood, S. J., Simmons, V.,Wild, G.C. 'Antiviral Properties of Garlic: In Vitro Effects of Influenza B, Herpes Simplex and Coxsackie Viruses' *Plant Medica* 460: Oct. 1985

IMPOTENCY

British Herbal Pharmocopoeia p 52, 1983

Kim, C., Choi, H., Kim, C.C. 'Influence of Ginseng on mating action of male rats' *Ann. J. Chinese Med.* 4: pp 163-8, 1970

INSOMNIA

British Herbal Pharmacopoeia pp 153-4, 225-6, 1983

Fitten, L.H. 'L-Tryptophan as a Hypnotic in Special Patients' *J. Am. Geriat. Soc.* 33:p 294, 1985

Mohler, H. 'Nicotinamide is a brain constituent with benzodiazepine-like actions' *Nature* 278: pp 563-65, 1979

MEMORY

Dysken, M.A. 'Review of recent clinical trials in the treatment of Alzheimer's Dementia' *Psychiatric Annals* 17 (3): p 178, 1987

Hindmarch, I 'The psychopharmacological effects of Ginkgo biloba extract in normal healthy volunteers' *Int. J. Clin. Pharmacol. Res.* 4: pp 39-43, 1984

King, R.G. 'Do raised aluminium levels in Alzheimer's Dementia cholinergic neuronal deficits?' *Med. Hypoth.* 14: pp 301-6, 1984

Muller, D 'Vitamin E in brains of patients with Alzheimer's Disease and Down Syndrome' *Lancet* 1: pp 1093-4, 1986

MENOPAUSE

British Herbal Pharmocopoeia p 37, 1983

Duke, J.A., Ayensu, E.S. Medicinal Plants of China (Reference Publication, 1985)

Finkler, R.S. 'The Effects of Vitamin E in the menopause' *J. Clin. Endocrin. Metabol.* 9: pp 89-94, 1949

Smith, C.J. 'Non-hormonal control of vaso-motor flushing in menopausal patients' *Chicago Med.* 7 March 1964

MENSTRUATION

Bettini, V. 'Effects of Vaccinium myrtillus anthocyanosides on vascular smooth muscle' *Fitoterapia* 55: pp 265-72, 1984

Butler, E.B., McKnight, E 'Vitamin E in the treatment of primary dysmenorrhoea' *Lancet* 1: pp 1844-47, 1955

Stuart, M.(ed) The Encyclopaedia of Herbs and Herbalism (Orbis Publishing, Bristol, 1979)

NIGHT VISION

Sala, D. 'Effect of Anthoyanoides on Visual Performance at Low Illumination' *Minerva Oftamol* 21: pp 283-5, 1979

Underwood, B. Vitamin A in Animal and Human Nutrition in the Retinoid (Academic Press, 1984)

OSTEOPOROSIS

Barzel, U.S. 'Acid loading and osteoporosis' *J. Am. Geriatrics Soc.* Sept. 1982

Draper, H.H., Scythes, C.A. 'Calcium, Phosphorous and Osteoporosis' *Fed. Proc.* 40(9): pp 2434-38, 1981

Hollingbery, P.W. 'Effect 'of Dietary Caffeine and Aspirin on Urinary Calcium and Hydroxyproline Excretion in Pre- and Menopausal Women' *Fed. Proc.* 44: p 1149, 1985

Worthington-Roberts, B. *Contemporary Developments in Nutrition* St Lewis, MO, CV, Mosby Co., 1981

PREGNANCY

Gold, S., Sherry, L. 'Hyperactivity, learning disabilities and alcohol' *J. Learning Disabilities* 17(1): pp 3-6, 1984

Laurence, K.M. 'Double-blind randomized controlled trial of folate treatment before conception to prevent recurrence of neural tube defects' *Brit. Med. J.* 282: p 1509, 1981

Mowrey Scientific Validation of Herbal Medicine (Keats Publishing, Conneticut, 1986)

O'Brien, P.M.S. 'The effect of dietary supplementation with linoleic acid and linolenic acid on the pressor response to antiotension 11: A possible role in pregnancy-induced hypertension' *British J. Clin. Pharmacol.* 19(3): pp 335-42, 1985

Smitheus, R.W. 'Apparent prevention of neural tube defects by periconceptional vitamin supplementation' *Arch. Dis. Childhood* 56: p 911, 1981

Sutton, R.V. 'Vitamin E in Habitual Abortion' *Brit. Med. J.* 4 Oct. 1958

Tolarovam, M. 'Periconceptional supplementation with vitamins and folic acid to prevent recurrence of cleft lip' *Lancet* 2: p 217, 1982

Truswell, A.S. 'Nutrition for pregnancy' *Brit. Med. J.* July, 1985

PMT

Barr, W. 'Pyridoxine supplements in the Pre-menstrual Syndrome' *Practitioner* 228: pp 425-7, 1984

Horrobin, D.F. 'The role of essential fatty acids and prostaglandins in the pre-menstrual syndrome' *J. Reprod. Med.* 28 (7): pp 465-68, 1983

Piesse, J.W. 'Nutritional Factors in the Pre-Menstrual Syndrome' *Int. Clin. Nutr. Rev.* 4: pp 54-81, 1984

TINNITUS

British Herbal Pharmacopoeia pp 41-2, 65-6, 1983

Browning, G.G. 'Blood viscosity as a factor in sensorineural hearing impairment' *Lancet* 1: pp 121-23, 1986

Dolev, E. 'Is magnesium depletion the reason for ototoxicity caused by aminoglycosides?' *Med. Hypotheses* 10(4): pp353-58, 1983

Vorberg, G. 'Ginkgo biloba extract (GBE): A long term study of chronic cerebral insufficiency in geriatic patients' *Clinical Trials J.* 22: pp149-57, 1985

VARICOSE VEINS

Fuji, T. 'The clinical effects of vitamin E on purpuras due to vascular defects' *J. Vitaminology* 18: pp 125-30, 1972

Spapiro, S. Spitzer, J.M. 'The Use of Cepevit (Abscorbic Acid plus 'P' Factors) in drug induced hypoprothrombinemia' *Angiology* 5: pp 64-71, 1954

INDEX

abortion 23, 106
abscesses 130
acid foods 7, 8, 24, 29, 66
acne 20, 21
ageing spots 21, 22
Agrimony Complex 68
Agropyron repens 128
AIDS 89, 91, 136
alcohol 10, 23, 79, 82, 120
alcohol foetal syndrome ... 106

alfalfa 124
alkaline foods 7, 8, 24, 66
allergies   12, 24, 68, 73, 83, 101, 109
Allium sativum 131
Aloe vera 124
aluminium 156
Alzheimer's Disease 26
American cranesbill 128
amyloidosis 22
anaemia 64, 129

analgesic 26, 34, 83, 129
Anethum graveolens 129
Angelica sinensis 129
angina 79, 133
aniseed 124
antibiotics 12, 50
antioxidants ... 22, 27, 31, 48, 143
antiviral 89
anxiety 135, 137
Apium graveolens 127
Apple Fibre Complex 120
Apricot E Oil 66, 70
Apricot Moisturising Creme . 70
Arctostaphylos uva-ursi 139
arteries 84
arteriosclerosis 50
arthritis 28, 125, 127, 129, 132
artichoke 132
Asclepias tuberosa 136
aspirin 26, 137
asthma ... 24, 30, 130, 132, 137
athletes 14, 31
Avena sativa 134
Avocado Night Creme 70
babies 32, 68
back pain 26, 33, 34
bad breath 35
barberry 125
bayberry 125
bearberry 125
bed sores 35
bedwetting 128
Berberis vulgaris 125
beta-carotene . 27, 28, 40, 102, 103
bethroot 125
Betonica officinalis 125
betony 125
BIO Ace 28, 32, 40, 52, 71, 91,
BIO C 36, 60, 61, 95,
BIO Chromium 88
BIO Zinc 43, 44, 110
bites 36, 124
blood pressure 6, 38, 78-81, 88,
131, 134
blueberry 125
boils 130, 138
boldo 125
bones........... 45, 46, 104, 128
bowel polyps 40

bran 40, 62
bronchitis 42, 132
bruises 43, 112
buckthorn 126
burns 43, 124
caffeine 50, 134
calcium 18, 44, 104
calcium phosphate 104
camphor 126
cancer 40, 47-49, 129
Candida albicans 33, 35, 50, 77, 89
Capsicum annuum 127
carbohydrate 2, 88
carbuncles 130
cardiovascular 38, 39
Cascara sagrada 126
Cassia senna 126
cataracts 22
catarrh 89, 104, 129, 132
cayenne 127
Celery Complex 29
chickweed 127
Chickweed Compound 110
chilblains 52
childbirth 135
children 53, 87, 106, 114
cholesterol 41, 45, 54, 85, 113, 130
Chondrus crispus 134
chromium 151
cigarettes 11, 56, 57, 84
Cinnamon Scrub 70
Cimicifuga recemosa 125
Cinnamomum camphora 126
cirrhosis 96
cobalt 152
Cochlearia amoracia 134
coffee 10, 50, 104, 120
Cola nitida 134
cold hands and feet 58
colds 28, 42, 61, 130
cold sores 59
Cold Tablets 111
colic 32, 129, 137
colitis 64, 65
Colon Care 60
comfrey 122, 127, 128
Comfrey Ointment 112
conjunctivitis 130, 132
constipation 61, 126, 127

contraception 13
convulsion 137
corn silk 128
couch grass 128
coughs 130
cracking skin 62
cramps 63
Crataegus oxyancanthoides   133
Crohn's Disease 65
Chronic Fatigue Syndrome ... 89
Cynara scolymus 132
cystitis 65, 128
cytotoxic blood test 24, 30
dandelion 128
dandruff 66
decoctions 123
dermatitis 110
Dermatone 110
depression 105, 130, 134
devil's claw 128
diabetes 67
diarrhoea 68, 128
digestion 10, 124, 131
Digestive Aid 93
dill 129
disaccharides 2
diuretic   75, 124, 126, 128, 133
dong quai 98, 129
Echinacea augustiflolia 130
eczema 110
Eczema Balm 110
elder flower 130
elimination diet 24, 57
Ephedra sinica 26, 122, 130
epilepsy 71, 136
Equisitum arvense 134
Eucalyptus globulus 130
Eugenia caryophyllata 127
Euphorbia hirta 130
Euphrasia offinalis 131
evening primrose oil 131
Evening Primrose Body Lotion ..
71
eyebright 131
flatulence 131
fasting 73
fats 3, 47, 75, 96
fatty acids . 48, 63-67, 109, 113, 115
fennel 131

fenugreek 131
feverfew 131
fibre 40, 41, 62, 69
fluid retention 74, 105, 116
fluorine 152
Foeniculum vulgare 131
gallbladder ...,.... 125, 126, 128
free radicals 31, 47, 48
gallbladder 75, 76, 78
gallstones 75, 76
Garlix 54, 56, 85
garlic .. 38, 77, 78, 85, 89, 114, 131
Gaultheria procumbens 132
Gentian lutea 132
ginger 132
gingseng 132
Ginkgo biloba 97, 113, 11
Globe artichoke 132
Gycyrrhiza glabra 134
golden seal 122, 132
gout 28, 78, 103
Grindelia robusta 133
Guaiacum officinale 133
haemorrhaging 132
hair 15, 21, 66,
halitosis 35
Harpagophytum procumbens 129
hawthorn 38, 79, 80, 133
hayfever 81, 82, 130
headache ... 26, 62, 67, 82, 100, 105, 125, 137
heart disease 38, 50, 54, 79, 80, 84-6
Heat Rub 112
hepatitis 86, 95, 134
Herbal Diuretic Formula 75
herpes 59, 86, 89,
hops 133
hormone imbalance 99, 129
horseradish 134
horsetail 133
Humulus lupulus 133
Hydrastis canadensis 132
hyperactivity 87, 106, 136
Hypericum perforatum 137
hypertension 38, 134
hypoglycaemia 88
immune system 28, 29, 61, 78, 89-91, 116
impotency 91

incontinence 137
indigestion 92, 135
influenza 28, 61, 78, 89
insomnia 92, 133, 135, 137
insulin 67
intermittent claudication 94, 95
iodine 152
Irish moss 134
iron 18, 153
jaundice 75
juniper 128, 134
Juniperus communis 134
kelp 134
kidneys 128, 133
kola 134
Lactobacillus acidophilus ... 33,
35, 50, 51, 92
legs 15, 96, 115
leukaemia 43
lime flowers 134
lips 14
lipoprotein 54
liquid extracts 123
liquorice 134
liver 23, 95, 96, 128, 134
lysine 19, 59
magnesium .... 153 phosphate
.... 114
Marrubium vulgare 133
marshmallow 65
Marshmallow Soap 71
Medicago sativa 124
Melaleuca alternifolia 139
memory 97, 131
menopause 45, 98, 104, 129
menstruation . 74, 98, 105, 125, 129
Mentha x piperita 136
Mentha spicata 137
metabolism 117, 131
methionine(DL-) 27
migraine 24, 82, 83, 100
milk thistle 23, 135
mineral 143, 152
miscarriage 106
monosaccharides 2, 106
morning sickness 107
mullein 135
multiple sclerosis .. 89, 90, 102
nails 15, 86, 120

nappy rash 33
nausea 114
neuralgia 26
Mineral 104, 107
night vision 73, 125
nutrition 1-19
oats 135
Oenothera biennis 131
oestrogen 98-100
olive oil 76, 135
osteoarthritis 28, 103, 135
osteoporosis 45, 104
palpitation 79
Panax ginseng 132
Passiflora incarnata .. 135, 137
peppermint 135
percolations 123
Peritone 62
Peumus boldus 125
phosphorous 154
Pimpinella anisum 124
Plantago psyllium 136
pleurisy 136
potassium 154
Polygala senega 137
polysaccharides 2
polyunsaturated 54
potassium 154
potassium chloride 109
potassium phosphate . 113, 114
potatoes 24
prednizone 64
pregnancy 13, 106
prescribed drugs 97, 108
PMT 12, 74, 105
PMT Formula 100, 105
prostate 65, 91, 108, 120
protein 3, 88, 104
psoriasis 136
raspberry 24, 30, 136
RAST 24, 30
Raynaud's Disease 58, 109
RDA/RDI 9, 14-19
reproduction 13, 106
Rhamnus cathartica 126
Rhammnus purshiana 126
rheumatism 26, 137
rheumatoid arthritis 28, 29, 109
rhubarb 136

172   *Index*

Rubus idaes 136
ringworm 139
St John's Wort 91, 137
salicin 26, 137
salt 5, 39, 74
Sambuccus nigra 130
Sarsparilla Complex 110, 13
scullcap 137
Scutellaria laterifolia 136
selenium 47, 154
septicaemia 130
Serenoa repens 137
silica 86
Silybum marianum 135
sinusitis 89, 109, 129, 131, 133
skin ... 14, 20, 62, 70, 109, 136, 143
sleep 93, 94
slippery elm 137
Smilax ornata 11, 104, 111
sodium 155
sore throat . 109, 111, 125, 137
spearmint 138
sprains 111
Stellaria media 127
stings 36
stomach ulcers ... 93, 106, 128, 137
strains 111
stress .... ii, vii, 12, 112
sugar 65, 88
Symphytum officinale 127, 128
Taraxum officinale 10, 50, 129
tea tree oil 139
thrush 50
Thuja occidentalis 139
thyme 139
Thymus vulgaris 139
thyroid 134
Tillia cordata 134
tinctures 123
tinea 137
tinnitus 109, 113
Tranquil Night Formula 92
Travel Calm Ginger ... 107, 115
travel sickness 114, 131
Trigonella foenum-graecum 131
Trillium erectum 125

tryptophan 93
ulcers 93, 95, 102, 124, 132, 142
Ulmus fulva 136
uva-ursi 139
urticaria 26
Vaccinium myrtillus 125
Valeriana officinalis 139
varicose veins 115
Verbascum thapsus 135
vertigo 113, 116,
viruses 42, 89-91, 129
vitamins — general 10-19
  A 144
  B1 (thiamin) 144
  B2 (riboflavin) 144
  B3 (niacin/nicotinic acid) 144
  B5 (pantothenic acid) ... 144
  B6 (pyridoxine) 145
  B12(cabalamin) 146
  B13 (orotic acid) 146
  B15 (pangamic acid) 146
  B17 (laetrile) 146
  biotin 147
  C (abscorbic acid) 148
  choline 147
  D 148
  E (tocopherol) 149
  F 149
  folic acid 145
  inositol 147
  K (menadine) 149
  P (flavonoids) 149
  PABA 148
  T............................. 150
  U 150
water 1, 29, 62, 117
warts 116, 134, 137
weight loss ... 85, 86, 87, 103, 116
weight loss diet 117, 119
white willow bark 140
Wild Nettle Shampoo 66
Witch Hazel Toner 70
wintergreen 140
Zea mays 128
zinc 18, 120, 155
Zingiber officinale 132